Grow Taller

Vitamins Your Body Needs to Get Taller Fast

(How to Be Taller Quickly and Easily With Simple Home Exercises)

Harold Waller

Published By **Darby Connor**

Harold Waller

Grow Taller: Vitamins Your Body Needs to Get Taller Fast (How to Be Taller Quickly and Easily With Simple Home Exercises)

ISBN 978-1-77485-537-9

No part of this guidebook shall be reproduced in any form without permission in writing from the publisher except in the case of brief quotations embodied in critical articles or reviews.

Legal & Disclaimer

The information contained in this ebook is not designed to replace or take the place of any form of medicine or professional medical advice. The information in this ebook has been provided for educational & entertainment purposes only.

The information contained in this book has been compiled from sources deemed reliable, and it is accurate to the best of the Author's knowledge; however, the Author cannot guarantee its accuracy and validity and cannot be held liable for any errors or omissions. Changes are periodically made to this book. You must consult your doctor or get professional medical advice before using any of the suggested remedies, techniques, or information in this book.

Upon using the information contained in this book, you agree to hold harmless the Author from and against any damages, costs, and expenses, including any legal fees potentially resulting from the application of any of the information provided by this guide. This disclaimer applies to any damages or injury caused by the use and application, whether directly or indirectly, of any advice or information presented, whether for breach of contract, tort, negligence, personal injury, criminal intent, or under any other cause of action.

You agree to accept all risks of using the information presented inside this book. You need to consult a professional medical practitioner in order to ensure you are both able and healthy enough to participate in this program.

TABLE OF CONTENTS

Introduction 1

Chapter 1: How Growth Happens Growth, Physiology, And Development Hormones 3

Chapter 2: Therapy Using Exogenous Gh 10

Chapter 3: Your Sleep Quality 19

Chapter 4: Eating As A Natural Method To Stimulate Hgh Secretion 25

Chapter 5: Exercise To Increase Growth: Basic Routines 36

Chapter 6: Stretching To Lengthen Muscles And Bones Day One 42

Chapter 7: Stretching To Strengthen Muscles And Bones Day Two 47

Chapter 8: Exercises To Get Taller 71

Chapter 9: Which Actually Stunts Growth? 80

Chapter 10: Additional Strategies To Control Height 83

Chapter 11: Genes And You 86

Chapter 12: Actors Subject To Growth. 107

Chapter 13: "Eat The Right Kinds Of Food 167

Conclusion 183

Introduction

An effective effort to get taller requires a combination of all three essential elements: Sato, exercise and adequate nutrition.

There are many other aspects that help you in getting taller, like your posture and sleep habits, but the three mentioned above are the most crucial ones to consider for a better height increase.

A typical person regardless of how tall he/she is, is likely to be taller by between 2 and 4 inches. What is the reason why most people are smaller than they are? It's because they aren't aware of how to maximize their potential. That's why we designed an approach to help maximise potential growth for people who aren't satisfied with their height. If you believe that growing higher will bring you benefits in your day life and actually want these advantages This program will bring you the best results. You must be able to believe in the work you're doing Believe in the results, and believe in what you're reading here.

Our approach has proved to the real world to be an effective method of growing. This method is effective even for people who haven't seen an increase in their growth over the last few years. In our research and trials with people from different age groups willing to experiment with our method, we discovered that even in the age range of 25-30 people can gain 1 to 4 inches! At 30 and beyond, there's the possibility of growing!

Satogrowth's programs and treatments will aid in improving your posture overall and grow.

Chapter 1: How Growth Happens Growth, Physiology, And Development Hormones

The first and most important thing is that we must understand the entire process of growth and everything related to it. It is true that our habits, lifestyle and the quality of our lives are all a part of the equation about the size we'll get.

Once, you were one cell that resulted from an fusion between two cells, that you received from your father and mother. It's pretty impressive growth given your current size isn't it? Seedlings develop to fully mature organisms. They grow other seeds as well.

What is the place where growth begins?

The simple answer is that you begin to grow from the moment of fertilization. The two cells of your father and mother join into one single cell and then division begins. Cells continue to divide to create organs, tissues and systems. Bones are also composed of dense, strong tissue.

Cell cycle

The term "cell cycle" is used to describe the continual division of cells as well as replacement. Cell cycles are crucial to human existence and serve two main functions to perform:

Growth and development

Keep your body healthy

We've observed the link between cell cycle and growth. But how do such cycles help keep your organism healthy? Let's start with the fact that we do not anymore are surrounded by the exact skin cells as you used to have four years ago.

Your cells are limited in number of divisions. This leads them to get older and eventually die after a certain time. This means that your body is constantly replacing cells with new cells. However, the number of replacements (cycles) is also restricted by DNA, which restricts the lifespan of every living thing.

Skin loses its elasticity and dies. Red blood cells die too. Every cell within our body requires replacement. However, since the human experience on Earth is just a moment in time it is inevitable that we will become tired, wrinkled and our organs and systems slowly cease to function.

However, let's not go for granted - it's a horrible thought for someone looking through this book looking for ways to get taller! There are many kinds of cells that are that are growing, dying, and then being replaced however this doesn't happen randomly.

There are special areas of our brain that are in charge different kinds of multiplication of cells.

Chemical and physiological processes

The growth hormone of animals (somatotropin called STH) is produced naturally by the pituitary anterior gland (also called the adenohypophysis). It is a tiny gland of the endocrine system about that is the size of peas that produce nine hormones.

Also, it regulates range of physiological processes, like:

Energy;

Balance of water;

Tissue repair;

Fat burn and metabolism;

Lactation;

Reproduction;

Stress

The hormones produced from the pituitary gland's anterior part manage the function of various important organs, tissues and glands.

The thyroid gland

Adrenal gland (which produces and releases adrenaline);

The gonads (sexual organs that make eggs and sperm, testes in males and ovaries in women);

Bones;

The liver

But it is important to note that the pituitary anterior gland does not function as the "boss" even though it appears to be. The reason is that it is controlled by the hypothalamus - the brain's small portion that is responsible for controlling metabolism as well as facilitating communication between the endocrine and nervous systems.

Other side effects of the growth hormone produced by the body

Immune system stimulation;

Protein synthesis stimulation;

Improvement in the function of the pancreas;

Aids in the retention of calcium (and thus the strengthening of bones);

Muscle mass is increased;

It stimulates the development of all organs in the body with the exception of the brain.

Contributes to the homeostasis process (our body's ability to keep internal balance by controlling various properties such as temperature or pH)

Growth hormone underproduction

The consequences of GH deficiencies are mostly influenced by the age of the patient. For children, GH deficiencies can cause diminution in height or even inability. Additionally, sexual maturation that is not complete and being overweight are usually linked to the same issue.

GH deficiency is uncommon for adults, however, generally speaking the most common symptom of

GH deficiency is pituitary tumors. Pituitary tumors are not cancerous benign tumors that attach to the pituitary gland.

People with low GH levels typically have greater body mass than muscles. They appear larger than they actually are, or to struggle with excess weight and obesity.

GH deficiency can be caused by genetic issues as well as congenital anomalies. In some instances the environment plays a significant part in the release of its hormones. A child who is raised in a dark, cramped space, and lacking fresh air may show signs for GH deficiency.

Growth hormone overproduction

Being deficient isn't a good thing But being overloaded isn't any better. GH excess can cause pituitary tumours (adenomas) comprised of somatotrophic cells inside the anterior pituitary gland.

Even if adenomas are slow-growing and are not harmful but they can get sufficient to put pressure on the optic nerve if untreated. This causes vision impairment and migraines. It can also influence the production of pituitary hormones in other ways.

Chapter 2: Therapy Using Exogenous Gh

There are a few things to keep in mind here:

The administration of exogenous GH (exogenous=not created by your body) for treatment isn't suggested, but it is an option last resort in small instances.

The administration of GH should be done cautiously and in tiny amounts to allow the progress of the drug to be observed and adverse effects to be efficiently controlled should they occur.

Always consult your physician prior to using any hormone-based treatments and only purchase hormone-based items from authorized retailers (pharmacies) only that are based on the prescription of your doctor.

The short stature of a person isn't always due to GH deficiency. GH supplements can also be prescribed to treat certain ailments that aren't caused by hormone imbalances, for instance:

The chronic renal condition;

Intrauterine growth retardation;

It is also known as Turner syndrome (a genetic disorder) whose manifestations include lymphedema and rudimentary reproductive system, sterility or amenorrhoea and obesity, as well as short height, hips are big, while waists are tiny, with poor vision, facial characteristics);

A condition known as Prader-Willi syndrome (a rare genetic disorder that causes the diminution of stature, a poor or ineffective sexual development in excess hunger, and insufficient muscular tone).

Common side effects

GH treatment options have been FDA certified for use in a small amount of patients that means they are generally safe to use in the areas where they are most needed and in the proper quantities. The most common side effects can include:

Carpal tunnel syndrome;

Joint pain, swelling and/or pain;

The risk of having diabetes may increase

Supplements, GH and the US law

There are a myriad of websites that sell diet supplements that contain herbs, vitamins and amino acids that are designed to boost GH production. They're legal in the sense that they claim to be dietary supplements , and consequently don't include the hormone themselves (exogenous GH is a drug that is not a dietary supplement).

Additionally there is a US law also prohibits supplement companies to promote or claim advantages to health (such for the treatment of specific illnesses and ailments) in connection with taking supplements. Additionally, advertisements must state that the benefits they claim to have, and that they aren't FDA certified.

Take a close examine what you're purchasing and stay away from sellers who sell obscure products. It is imperative to consult your doctor prior to using any type of supplement. If your doctor is in agreement that you should not purchase supplements on the internet. Drug stores are the most secure and reliable sources.

Can You Be Taller? Factors Influencing Height

Do you have a family that is taller than you? Do you think that your lifestyle and lifestyle may influence your growth? Now, we'll look at the possibilities, take a look and see if any of them is appropriate for your particular situation.

Genetics

We're all exhausted of hearing that. You're part of a family of people who aren't tall and so why should you be more taller than the rest of them? Genes have an important role to play regarding this height issue however that does not mean that your bones won't be able to stretch if you adhere to your routine of stretching and remain positive.

In the worst scenario the genes will only hinder your ability to gain height however, it is not will it be impossible. If you put in the effort and time you'll be able to gain an inch or two and become the most tallest person on your own family! It is hoped that this won't transform you into a sort or"black sheep...

Extra-nutriental... maybe it's not...

The growth rate is directly linked to the food you're fed as a young child. The food you eat for your child must be rich in calcium, protein, and vitamins. Protein is important to develop muscle strength and build strength. Vitamins and calcium are essential to build strong and long-lasting bones. It is also important to maintain a healthy immune system.

If your diet was focused on junk food, it's no reason why you haven't developed to all of your "capabilities"! In addition, you may struggle with excess weight and high cholesterol.

The most fortunate of us can stay within our normal weight range even though we eat junk foods on a regular basis This is due to the good genes and a fast metabolism can slow down or even stop weight increase. But, there are plenty of young and slim children that eat just unhealthy foods... What's the difference?

Genes. Genes control the behavior of our bodies even the smallest small of details. Being overweight doesn't necessarily mean you consume too much healthy food It's just that you're eating excessively. There are people who add weight (quantity) and still be unnourished from an nutritional (quality) perspective.

As you prepare to grow more taller, changing your diet is likely to be the first thing you'll need to think about. Keep in mind that I'll go over the nutritional aspect later within the text.

Physical and postural activity

Do you spend a lot of your time seated or at the computer? If yes then your spinal column (spine) might be experiencing immense pressure. The length of your spine is comparable to your height. Therefore, any strain that is prolonged will stop it from growing , and will add noticeable inches in your daily measurements.

Furthermore, not participating in physical exercise can cause mild muscle atrophy (as muscles no longer in good shape). If your musculoskeletal body doesn't take part in regular physical activities it won't strengthen or develop.

Do not sleep at night

It has been proven scientifically that the hormone that causes human growth is produced in large amounts and is released efficiently in the nighttime. Biologically and genetically human beings are designed to function as diurnal (carry various activities during the day, and thus recharge batteries in the evening).

It is vital for teens and children to get enough sleep - approximately 8 hours per day, with the ideal time being between 10-11 pm until 6-7 am. Growth hormone production is at its peak at midnight, therefore it is ideal to avoid going to bed after 11 pm.

Hormonal imbalance

The endocrine system can be extremely sensitive and not something you can play around with. Hormones are responsible for regulating the body's functions and processes and if they are tampered by (e.g. begins to produce hormones that are too high or low) and the whole system ceases to function properly.

Certain hormone treatments may reduce or even stop growth. If this is the case ensure that you confirm your hormone levels with the most qualified doctor you locate. A small error in the diagnosis or prescription could cause you to lose your entire life.

Starting Off: Getting Proper Sleep

The greatest amounts of somatotropin are released during the night. It is therefore essential for teenagers and children to get up early and to sleep for at least 8 hours every day to ensure optimal development and to encourage growth spurts.

It's been proved scientifically that exercising and sleeping are the most efficient natural stimuli for GH production. This is the simplest way to go You don't need to drink some strange cocktail or pay for costly (and likely useless) treatment options.

Perseverance, free will and a structured plan are the top traits you need to be working on if you want to increase your height. Try to focus on the long-term (well in fact, lasting) ...) adjustments), stick to your plan , and outcomes will be visible quickly.

What time should I be able to sleep?

The most hGH-rich levels will be released after 60-90 minutes of sleeping when you go to sleep at 11 pm or earlier. The optimal time for releasing hGH is at or near midnight. This is how nature operates.

I stopped growing at the age of 15 that's the exact year that I began sleeping around 3-4 am. This habit lingered for many years and, after all the damage I'd done to myself, I kept asking myself why I did not increase my height beyond 5".

Naps

When you're an athlete, or someone who is very active do not be afraid to take a time off throughout the daytime. HGH can also be secreted during naps in the day, if you're keen on exercising.

Exercise and sleep as powerful personal stimuli, but in these conditions, taking naps in the day makes use of the force of both! What wouldn't be amazing? We're just going to have to move you... and you'll learn everything you need you need to know about exercise later in the book.

Chapter 3: Your Sleep Quality

You're not alone the positive effects of a restful night's sleep can be lost in the absence of relaxation and peace. Make a plan for your sleeping time. Turn off any electronic device, including telephones and intercoms.

I guarantee that your phone's ringtone is the last thing you'd like to be hearing during the most intense phases of your priceless sleeping hours. Also, getting up with that kind of a ringtone is painful, so I suggest turning off everything Better safe than sorry.

Don't be a fool and assume that nobody will ever call you to get you up. You don't have the luxury of knowing. If someone on the planet has your number, then you could be reached at any time any time, from any time. You are entitled to be in the privacy of your home, so make use of your right to privacy!

Check that your bed couch is comfortable enough . an inflatable mattress and soft, clean sheets work wonders. Peace and freshness will help you sleep in just a few minutes. You can opt for silk or cotton sheets. Mmm, comfy...

If it takes you longer than 15-30 minutes before falling asleep, you may be experiencing some sort of issue. Problems? Worries? Concerns? It is time to find ways to get rid of these. Speak to a trusted person you trust or seek expert help to get them off your head and off your chest.

Keep in mind that insomnia and nightmares can develop into medical conditions when they are experienced frequently. Sometimes, talking to your doctor about the issue is the best method to figure out how you can achieve mental tranquility and sleep at ease. The professionals are here to assist and assist you, so don't hesitate consult them.

How inadequate nutrition steals off Inches

It's time to get to a significant improvement and change your eating routine. The first step is to examine what we're not required to do if we aren't looking to be unsatisfied and short...

In the night, eating carbs

We've observed that 85 percent of the amount of hGH is secreted at evening, while you sleeping. We also know that it regulates metabolism and metabolism rates for fat burning. So far, all well, but what does it have to do with late-night and carb-rich eating?

Consuming foods high in carbs can cause the levels of insulin to rise. Glucose is pumped directly to the tissues of your body and insulin works to help keep your blood sugar in the normal range.

The issue is that hormone secretion is impeded by elevated insulin levels and higher levels of hGH decrease insulin secretion (this is the reason why people who are treated with exogenous hGH suffer with a greater risk of developing diabetes). The hormones hGH and insulin are antagonists.

If insulin blocks hGH production Imagine the harm you'd result from eating a dinner filled with HGH inhibitors before sleep (on on a regular basis and, naturally). Children require extra supervision and must be aware of the consequences at the age of.

Furthermore, insulin levels that are high can also trigger fat accumulation. In the event of the inhibition of hGH muscle recovery could be in a slow manner and the bone mineral density could reduce. The most effective way to combat this is to reduce your intake of carbs by avoiding foods that are high in carbs altogether.

The following food items:

White bread and all other products made from refined grains, such as rice, pasta, or pasta;

Baked products;

Sweets, such as drinks that are sweet.

Mineral and vitamin deficiencies

Your bones require calcium, vitamins , and other minerals in order to grow tall and robust. If your diet is deficient in these three elements and you don't get the height your gene code requires, or, even more your risk of suffering from fractures increases.

As time passes, a decrease in mineral density leads to osteoporosis. it's when the hard dense bone tissue turns porous and spongy. It can mean only one thing: extreme discomfort and the risk of fractures.

While osteoporosis tends to be found in people who are 40 and 50, unhealthy diets could cause it earlier, or make it considerably more difficult to manage during your senior years. Additionally, if the bone marrow is robust and dense, the bones are more likely to increase in size because they don't want to stay excessively thick!

Fat stuff

There are a lot more things to discuss in terms of fats. For starters, proteins and vitamins are way more healthy than fat. While we may need fat to live it can be a problem when we consume more calories than we require and then store the excess.

A sagging appearance, low self-esteem heart problems and heart diseases are just some of the lasting negative effects of eating excessively or having the diet that's largely made up of fat-based foods. Weight gain is so easy to gain and difficult to shed.

In addition, being overweight places extra stress over your spinal column as well as intervertebral discs. This hinders growth and serves as an increased risk for herniated discs, deformities and disproportions (an insufficient upper body to lower weight ratio).

Protein deficiency

Muscles are made up of proteins. In certain instances, if your bones grow longer while your muscle mass remains at the exact same level, then you're likely to appear thin or perhaps not athletic enough. Get plenty of protein! Build your strength to your new size!

Chapter 4: Eating As A Natural Method To Stimulate Hgh Secretion

The next topic will be the foods that are known to increase the production of hGH. It is not necessary to think about supplements or other drastic methods, since nature already provides all the tools to alter how our brain functions... and in the most safe, secure method.

We will concentrate on two major aspects of the diet:

The most important food items are: when, what and when

Bonus: natural hGH cocktail!

The body's nutritional requirements are the most crucial food items

Let's look at vitamin B12, vitamin A and vitamin B6. Vitamin A Vitamin A, Vitamin B6 along with vitamin B12 are among the most well-known growth-promoting vitamins that are available. These are available from:

Liver;

Kidney;

Fish oil (also extracted from the liver, plus vitamin K as well as Vitamin D);

A variety of meat (chicken pork, ham - also high in B1 vitamins, including beef);

Dairy products (especially eggs and milk)

All of these should be eaten in moderate amounts. It is recommended to eat meat at least at least two times per week. Consuming too much results in an increase in weight and may cause problems with cholesterol. Take care!

Another nutrient that we should pay attention to is fiber. Fiber aids in building muscle mass, which allows you to perform your routine of exercise without difficulty without becoming exhausted or painful. Fiber comes from:

Cereal;

Oatmeal;

Some fruits (banana, avocado, apples).

Strong bones will never be deficient in Vitamin C. There are numerous sources of vitamin C in food The most significant are:

Citrus fruits like citrus fruits like lemons and oranges that can be eaten fresh;

Wild berries;

Cauliflower;

Cabbage;

Tomatoes;

Potatoes

Vitamin C is a vitamin that has no effect if the food items containing it aren't longer in good condition or are stored at the temperature of room for a long time!

Vitamin D is obtained from dairy and milk products or just by taking a stroll in the sunlight. Vitamin D is created naturally by our bodies when exposed to sunlight. If your region isn't able to let sunlight through, you can take it as a compliment and drink a glass fresh milk each day!

Another vital mineral is vitamin F, that is found in:

Nuts;

Seeds (sunflower seeds, pumpkin seeds);

Oil from the sunflower;

Vegetable oil

Be wary of nuts - they're very calorific So, limit your consumption to no more than a handful in a day. Be aware of the oily and fried items. However, this doesn't mean you need to eliminate oil from your home however, you should try to avoid frequent consumption.

A word on supplementation...

Supplements are designed to help support your diet and increase the intake of certain nutrients. They're not an alternative for eating a balanced diet. Each supplement should be taken with caution and only if your doctor has instructed you to take it.

The minerals you require

You may have noticed, calcium is first ingredient on the list. It is not possible to sustain growth without calcium. The best calcium sources are meat and milk which are followed by soybeans, dried beans dried vegetables, sardines and dry beans.

Magnesium is among the essential minerals that are essential to health. Be sure to get enough magnesium from

Apples;

Figs;

Grapefruit;

Lemon;

Seeds, nuts and other seeds.

Fluoride and iodine can both be present in seafood. They play a significant role in the strengthening of bones together with calcium. Fluoride can make your teeth clear and strong.

Iron is essential for bone strength and helps to ensure the best blood circulation. It's found in many meats, but keep the moderation of consumption in your head. It isn't a good idea to have excessive iron in your body in the end.

It's true, chlorine is also crucial for health and well-being. It is usually found in table salt and along with table salt is sodium, which is a crucial mineral component. Don't over-exaggerate when it comes to salt, however - the tiny quantities used to add flavor to your meals are perfect.

Other minerals that are important to take into consideration are:

The mineral phosphorus (improves memory; it is present in the fish meat as well as fish oil);

Potassium;

Sulphur;

Zinc

The Natural Growth Hormone Drink

Drink this drink every day, after your workouts in the morning and after dinner. The ingredients are as follows:

One medium-sized tomato

Amount of 80g cabbage (white or red)

The beans weigh 80 grams (remove the skin)

You can also replace broad beans with:

Fava beans

Fresh green beans

Supplements with L-Dopa (remember to consult your physician first)

Method of preparation and method of preparation and

Mix the raw ingredients into blender. In case the mixture is thick enough, you can add water to make it more palatable. Additionally, you can include some sugar to improve the flavor, if needed.

The drink is best consumed 30-60 minutes after workouts in the morning and evening, and exercise. It's fine to consume the entire thing in one sitting If you're able, however avoid overindulging if you feel it's too excessive for you. Keep to half the amount in the morning and leave the rest for later in the evening.

What are these ingredients?

Cabbage is a great source of L-glutamine.

The tomato is a major source of gamma aminobutyric acid.

Broad beans contain a lot of L-Dopa.

Your levels of hGH are likely to increase by 300% following the consumption of this drink.

Exercising: General Instructions as well as Warnings

This is perhaps the most crucial part of the plan. Sleeping and eating well are vital to the process, however without exercise the body, there are no results that can be expected.

This is due to on the one hand, physical exercise can boost the production of hGH. However by focusing on certain types of workouts can extend and lengthen your bones and muscles. It's an incremental process, naturally therefore, you need to remain consistent.

The focus will be on stretching exercises and other activities to increase flexibility. Before we start it is important to be aware that these exercises are not to be performed in a random manner There are a set guidelines must be followed.

Lifting weights is FORBIDDEN

If you are looking to boost natural growth, refrain from lifting weights or any other type of strength-training. Heavy weights and doing work against weights in general will stress your spine, and throw off intervertebral discs.

Alongside the negative effects on the height of your body, weight lifting could cause hernias in the absence of supervision by a trained professional. However, if you are a fan of weightlifting take it up when your goals for growth have been attained.

A quick note about losing weight

The process of working against your body mass is similar to lifting weights but it's your own weight which can't be altered within a matter of weeks or days. If you're overweight or obese, lose the extra weight before beginning this exercise program to achieve outcomes.

Are you up to take on this physically?

Consult a doctor before doing one of the exercise routines, in particular the stretching exercises that are more difficult. We do not wish to cause injury to yourself because of a(n) (un)known health issue which could hinder these exercises from being completed smoothly.

Be fair

Yes, I would like you to remain consistently. Yes, I would like you to challenge yourself. But, you need to be aware of your limits and stay away from over-stressing your body.

Don't sit for long periods of time performing these exercises, or move into more challenging routines in case you're not prepared. Change is gradual and follows natural progression. You must push yourself, but in an a rational, sensible manner.

Beware of strains, soreness, and fatigue. It's better to exercise every day for 15 minutes instead of working for hours and not being able complete anything else throughout the week. Your body requires regularity and rhythm.

I suggest fifteen minutes of exercise each day. If you're confident that you're prepared you can go in for 30 minutes. Don't skimp steps and complete the warm-up exercises in the beginning even after you've completed your first week's exercises.

Materials

You'll need a mat , or a surface that is rough and has enough space to keep from getting injured.

Don't do the exercises in your bedroom because the mattress is too soft and bouncy. It will hinder your effectiveness. Certain exercises require a wall, chairs or a piece of furniture to help you.

Chapter 5: Exercise To Increase Growth: Basic Routines

The fundamental exercises should be performed within the first week in the course. I recommend that you do these exercises two times a morning: when you get up and then right after going to sleep. There's also a rationale to do this.

The vertebral column is stretched when you sleep, and it compresses throughout the daytime. Engaging in the exercises that introduce you to your body before you go to bed encourages the natural decompressing process and ensures that the spine is given the most stretch. Similar results occur when you perform the exercises just after you get up.

Exercise #1

Lay lying on the back. Your legs are slightly extended as you're able to hold your arms straight and raising your head.

Get your legs moving as long as you can.

Release.

Get your arms stretched out the length you are able to.

Release.

You can twist and rotate your body to the sides, while taking note of any potential injuries. The movements should be soft and fluid.

Exercise #2

Begin by lying onto your stomach.

Relieve your muscle tension.

Lift your legs and straighten them with your back to the ceiling.

Relax your arm and support the waist with them because your spine has to lift off the floor and your weight needs support in a certain way.

Make sure your legs are in an even (90 degrees) angle to the floor.

Continue to hold that position for couple of seconds.

Bend your knees, then begin to rotate your legs into the air like you're riding on a bicycle, as illustrated in the image below.

This rotary motion is expected to last around 1 minute.

Exercise #3

This exercise ensures that vertebrae and neck joints are also stretchy and flexible.

Make sure you sit up with the back in a straight position.

Make use of your arms to help hold yourself up by placing your hands in the ground, just a few inches from your body.

Make sure you rotate your head clockwise then turn it counterclockwise to prevent dizziness.

Be sure to extend your neck as far as you can during these movements It is also important to lengthen your neck!

Exercise #4

Spread your arms out laterally, at 90 degrees with the walls of your room.

Try to extend your arms backwards as far as you can. This will stretch and warm those arm muscles.

Rotate your arms ten times.

Shake them around.

Repeat this 10 times in the opposite direction.

Exercise #5

This exercise is divided into two sections.

Begin by standing straight, with your legs spread apart.

Your palms should be extended, and should be facing the wall that is in front of you.

Move your hands forward to lengthen muscles and bones, and loosen joints.

In both directions, reach out.

Even if you need to stretch as far as you can do not overdo it. Do not force yourself to do it, as injuries and strains are not part of the program.

The second part...

Keep your original place.

Turn your body to the left and right, then move as far as you are able to.

Repeat for 60 seconds.

Then, place your hands and place them behind your head and tilt for another 60 minutes.

Exercise #6

The exercise is performed in three phases.

Place yourself on the wall in front of it.

Reach as close as you can (this involves putting your body with it).

Make sure your feet are on the floor.

Raise your arm.

As high as you are able to.

Once you have reached the maximum height that you can extend to, keep your posture for a minimum of 10 seconds.

Lower your body gradually to the initial position.

Repeat this 10 times.

In the second installment...

Do not lower your arm, and rotate it 90 degrees.

Now, you are sitting with your elbow in front of the wall.

Repeat the stretching process until the height you can reach is at your highest then hold your position for about 10 seconds.

Repetition this process five times.

Turn sides and stretch once more.

Repeat five times more.

The third part...

Place your back against the wall.

Place both arms over your head.

You can stretch as far as you are able to.

If the maximum height is attained, hold the position for a period of 10 to 15 seconds.

Repetition this process five times.

Chapter 6: Stretching To Lengthen Muscles And Bones Day One

This chapter introduces some stretching movements that should be practiced in conjunction with the introduction exercises. The most effective time to incorporate them into your routine is to do these two times a day just after the exercise routine that was described in the previous chapter.

I'll walk you through fifteen of these exercises. Don't worry, you don't need to perform all of them in the same day. The exercises should be spread out over three days and be repeated over a period of 3 weeks (weeks 4 - 5).

Exercise #1

Get a chair and put it in your face.

One foot should be moved backwards away from the backrest of the chair.

Use the backrest to hold your arms up.

Take one leg off and move the opposite leg forwards, up to the ceiling, and gently leaning toward the front.

Lift this leg to the highest you are able and hold it throughout 10-20 seconds.

Repeat the exercise with your other leg.

Do this approximately 10 times per leg.

Exercise #2

Relax on your back.

One leg folds and then you move it towards your chest.

Pull your knee with your fingers and pull it towards your body.

Stop pulling your knee when it is in contact with your neck.

Keep that position for couple of seconds.

Release slowly and then return to the starting position.

Switch legs and complete these steps again.

Repeat this 10 times for each leg.

Exercise #3

Make sure your posture is in the right place.

Raise both hands above your head.

Reach up as high as you are able.

Do your best to keep your toes on while stretching.

Keep this position for approximately 1 minute if you're performing this exercise the very first time. It's best to aim for 2 minutes for the third time, but you shouldn't extend the time beyond three minutes otherwise you'll strain your muscles too long.

Exercise #4

Part One

You can lie on the floor on your stomach.

Put your arms and place them behind your back.

While not benting your knees and bending your knees, lift your upper body and lower lower body simultaneously.

These types of exercises are also referred to by the name of "Supermans". It's not necessary to do as much as the illustration above. A little bit of improvement every day is fine.

You can now move your body forward and backwards for a couple of minutes, while in this posture.

Repetition five times.

Part two

In the same position, spread your arms out in the direction of your body.

Lift your leg to the highest you can , and remain in the air for 20-30 seconds.

Switch legs.

Repeat this five times for each leg.

Exercise #5

Get up and extend your arms over your head.

Turn your upper body to the side and get as deeply into the exercise as you are able to.

Repeat ten times more (a left-right couple is counted as one).

Have a moment to rest , and repeat this again ten times.

Chapter 7: Stretching To Strengthen Muscles And Bones Day Two

On the second day, this program is a little more challenging However, do not worry about it the exercises will appear simpler once you are used to them over the long term.

Exercise #1

The exercise is designed to stretch spinal muscles and has been proven to be efficient in stimulating growth however, like any exercise that places your vertebrae to work, it must be performed with care to prevent injuries.

Lay down on your back and relax.

Place your palms on the floor, and stretch your knees.

Then gently lift your body towards the sky, as if were bending your hips in a slow movement.

Your body weight must now rest on your shoulders as well as your toes.

Slowly lower yourself to the original pose.

Repeat this ten times.

Exercise #2

Choose a comfortable chair, set it against a wall to provide support and then lie down.

You can extend diagonally, while keeping your spine as straight as you can.

The only areas of your body that will be in contact with the chair are your thighs and shoulders.

If you take a close look at the picture above, you will observe that the backrest of this chair is high, hindering you from performing the exercise in a 100% efficient manner (at the correct angle).

Maintain your body as rigid and straight as you can.

Continue to hold that position for couple of seconds.

Your body is folded up.

Move your chest forward, and lift your knees upwards like the picture above.

Utilize your arms to push your knees against your chest.

Repeat this exercise five times.

Exercise #3

Make sure you stand up with your feet away from each other (about 1 foot).).

As you rest your hands on your legs while holding your legs, bend your upper body upwards as you slide your fingers down.

Knees should not be bent (well this is a little too hard!).

The hamstrings should be getting stretched out and hurting. Do not worry about it and continue.

Then, let your hands go then lower them and ensure that your palms remain perfectly flat on the floor.

Exercise #4

Get up to a two feet away of the wall.

As long as you keep your lower body in a straight line and straight, bend your back until your fingers touch the wall. You could be used to help support your body weight.

Expand the space between you and your wall a couple of inches every day you do this workout (3 or 6 inches would be sufficient).

Repeat this exercise seven to ten times.

Exercise #5: bent forward lunge

Relax and stand up with your feet spaced apart.

You can move one leg forward while benting your knee while simultaneously.

The leg should be extended behind your body , but do not bend the knee.

As far forward as you can, without lifting your rear leg.

Keep it for five seconds.

Repeat the exercise five times, and then change legs and begin again.

Utilizing Stretching to Strengthen Muscles and Bones Day Three

Day three demands some extra effort.

Exercise #1

Get up and place your feet wide apart.

Begin to sink down to a full squat It's like sitting down on a chair that you can imagine.

Don't let your hips fall below the knee level. This is very harmful for your knees.

Your knees should be bent at 90 degrees.

Put your arms up in your face.

Do this 10 times.

Exercise #2

Relax and put your feet in the furniture (usually the couch or bed).

Maintain your lower body straight and remain still.

Revolve your torso clockwise, ten times.

Give yourself a moment and begin revolving clockwise over and over, 10 times.

Repeat it ten times in total.

Exercise #3

Make sure you stand up with your feet wide apart.

Place your hands to your head.

Join your hands to your sides and move them to the side.

Place your fingers on the floor.

If you are able to do it quickly, try using your hands instead.

Repeat 10 times.

You can increase the difficulty of this exercise by bringing your feet in a row.

Repeat 10 times. Repeat the process for a further ten times.

Exercise #4

Relax on your back.

Lift your arms over your head.

Then, raise your back to the highest point you can and as long as you're at ease.

Continue to work until your body's can be supported only by your heels and shoulders only.

The height of the arch each time you complete the exercise.

Repetition five times.

Exercise #5

Make sure you stand up with your feet at shoulder width.

Put your hands to your neck. Your right and left forearms should be in a straight line and your elbows should point forward.

Move forward, while keeping the spine in a straight line.

Try to reach your knees by bending your elbows.

Do not stretch too far and don't let your hands to press against your neck.

More advanced exercises

It's here the weeks from five to nine. This could be the most difficult portion in terms of exercise but it's also one of the most difficult and gorgeous. Be sure to do these exercises along with the other exercises mentioned in the earlier sections.

I'll now demonstrate 10 new exercises. You can choose five exercises to practice every day, along with the other scheduled exercises.

In the event that you have to perform these exercises twice a day, you could do five exercises in the morning and five at night instead of doing the same five exercises twice in a day. It's up to you.

Here are the final 10 exercises to be performed beginning in on the fifth week of this month...

Exercise #1

Get straight.

Put your hands behind the head (NOT over your head).

Make use of the hands of your fingers to press to the inside of your head, and then use your neck muscles stop it.

Do not release this tension and gently shift your head as far forward as is possible.

When your chin rests on your chest, slowly and gradually release the tension.

Repeat 10 times.

Stop for a few minutes and repeat the process 10 times.

Exercise #2

Get straight.

Place your hands to your back.

Secure your thumbs.

Your shoulders should be shifted back as far as is possible.

Lift your shoulders as high as you can.

Reduce your shoulders as far as is possible.

Imagine drawing circles using your shoulders. Then, you begin to move the circles in a rotary fashion.

Repeat this 10 times clockwise and 10 times counter-clockwise.

We've only described one set. Do 6 to 10 sets.

Exercise #3

Make sure you stand up and put your left foot forward.

The left leg must be straight and straight.

Your left arm should be extended on the same side, with your face straight towards the future.

Turn your left knee to the left and move your upper body downwards until your hands reach the floor.

Are you able to touch the floor with your entire area of your palm?

Go one move further and attempt to touch your head on the floor. It's not possible, but the effort itself will extend your back.

Repeat this 10 times.

Switch sides and repeat the process 10 times more.

Exercise #4

Make sure you stand up and put your feet together.

Spread your arms above your head.

Extend your arms upwards as far as you can.

Lift your feet up and continue to stretch your arms and upper body.

Then look up and hold the same position for five to ten seconds.

Repeat this ten times.

Exercise #5

Get up and place your feet at shoulder width.

Your hands rest between your hips.

Move forward, and then touch your right foot's toes with your left hand.

Slowly straighten yourself and then return to your initial posture.

Then bend forward, and finally make sure your left foot is in contact using your right hand.

As of now, everything is one. Repeat this nine times.

Don't get discouraged if aren't able to touch your feet the very first time. If you keep doing this exercise then you'll reach that point within a couple of weeks.

Exercise #6

Place your feet on the floor.

Stretch your legs out towards the front, and maintain your spine straight.

Put your hands on the hips.

Spread your hands outward and make sure your toes are touching while stretching your upper body.

Do this 5 times.

Then move your legs couple of inches apart, and then try again. Next, you can make sure your right foot is in contact with your left hand, and then reverse.

Repeat this process for five more times.

Exercise #7

Place your feet on the floor.

Your knees should be bent at 45 degrees.

Make sure your back is straight.

Put your hands behind your neck.

Turn your body sideways 5-10 times.

Now , try to align your right knee to your left elbow, and in reverse, as you twist.

The two movements are counted as one. You can also do four more.

Some people might find this workout too simple. If this is the scenario you can try to straighten your legs slightly. What do you feel like today?

Exercise #8

Lay down on your back and relax.

Your legs should be raised to the sky and hold your legs in a straight position.

Set your legs apart (as as you can) without having your knees bent.

Rejoin them and then start crossing them (as as you can). Imagine your legs as like a giant piece of string!

Repeat the exercise 10 times.

Pause for a moment and repeat this 10 times.

Exercise #9

Lay down on your back and relax.

Raise your legs in a vertical position.

Make sure you place your legs on your head like you were planning to get them back up.

Put your feet down on the floor, only a few inches away from your forehead.

Keep your legs straight , and remain in this position for 5-10 minutes.

Repeat this exercise 5 times.

Don't overdo it or strain yourself if you fail to make it the first time. Your strength and flexibility will increase with time.

Exercise #10

This activity is more complex, since you'll require advanced equipment or something similar that you could make at home.

In all cases it must be (or look like) the pull-up bar you're using that is sturdy enough, secure and securely fixed to hold your weight. Additionally, the pull-up bar needs to be at least one feet higher than the height of your body.

It is possible to ask an instructor to assist or assist you in accessing an elite gym. This is exactly what I did, and I believe it's the most secure and most reliable choice.

I would visit the fitness center to concentrate on cardio and at the end of each session I would stay longer to complete this workout using the pull-up bar.

Here's the information you'll need to know:

Jump up and grab the bar.

Secure it with your hands and move it both ways.

Take a break when your hands are tired and take a brief break.

Repeat the process 3-5 times.

I would recommend gentle movements - your hands will get tired and you'll not remain able to grip the bar for long enough to achieve outcomes.

Making use of Hypnosis to boost the Growth Process

The immense potential of hypnosis is frequently left unnoticed or unconsidered. Have you ever observed that belief in something results in you achieving the goal? It's a matter of psychological understanding and mastering it isn't an simple task.

A happy mind with an unfit body...

The connection between the mind and body isn't an all-or-nothing road. Your brain communicates with the proper nerves. However the same nerves also provide a feedback back to your brain.

Some examples of this feedback include the discomfort you feel when touching something warm, or that bizarre sensation that you'd feel if were outside in a shirtless winter. The skin's thermal receptors are directly linked to nerves and pathways.

Can you increase your growth through hypnosis?

There have been exceptional instances of people who "dissolved" tumors using their mental power, telling themselves they were healthy. The human brain can go well beyond the limits of its capabilities and we just need patience, time and faith.

Your brain has all the communication channels in order to "summon" growth hormones, making growth feasible at any stage or the age of. It is only necessary to be certain of one thing prior to you start.

There is a place in your heart that you have to believe in and be and firmly convinced that you'll grow since your mind is the sole responsible for this. Hypnosis is merely an intermediary between your body and mind which is the key to the full potential and power of your self.

You'll need to do for weeks, or months before you can get ability to master it. When you're on your own there is no voice that can guide your steps, and no other thing or piece of "reality" to grasp on to.

It's likely that you don't know what it feels to be hypnotized this moment, and the first time you'll achieve it successfully, you won't even be conscious up until the moment the time you "wake awake". This is why it is important to learn first.

This kind of hypnosis comes with four distinct stages:

Relaxation

Being relaxed physically allows your mind to enter an euphoric state. You should ensure that you have enough time to go through the entire session on weekends or in tranquil evenings are perfect. Relaxation should be a natural thing - don't make it happen by force.

Get away from any distractions and head to the quiet of your room. Relax on a bed recliner or sofa, as all your body needs to be able to rest in a comfortable way. Wear loose, comfortable clothes such as PJs or a dress gown.

Now, we will concentrate on the way you breathe as this is the most important step to attaining the sleep-like state.

You can place one finger on top of your chest and the other lies on your belly.

Do not try to alter your breathing rate at this moment. Just observe the hand that is rising when you breathe. If your abdomen raises then it's because you're breathing from your diaphragm, or, if you breathe through your chest.

Concentrate on breathing from your diaphragm. Take a deep breath through your nose and then slowly exhale by mouth. No sudden moves.

Make a tinny sound when you exhale through your mouth, something that sounds similar to "whoosh". Concentrate on the peace and peace that is triggered by this sound. It is quite similar to the sound of windor a relaxing calm sound like a sigh.

Inhale, exhale, and focus on the tranquility of the sound. Get ready to relax your muscles.

Progressive relaxation shows the connection between your body and your mind If you're stressed out, your muscles will get strained and become tight. But it also reveals that we can ease our minds by gradually relaxation of our muscles.

When you breathe out and in visualize that all tension has gone away, and that every muscle within your body is completely at peace, relaxed, and free of tension. Relax and tighten every part of your body , in the order listed below (you can keep a recording and play it back during the exercise):

Toes

Knees

Right leg. Relax your right leg fully and sinking into the soft, comfy mattress.

Left leg

Buttocks

Lower back

Stomach

Rib cage. Now you feel your lower body completely free from any tension.

Your shoulders should be pushed forward and back, then let your shoulders relax.

Imagine using your left arm. Make your fist. Lock your upper arm. Release. Then tighten the entire arm. Release.

Think about your left arm. Make your fist. Then tighten your upper arm. Release. Secure the entire arm. Release.

Relax your jaw and then release.

Keep your mouth open for about 2 seconds before you allow it to close.

The Grimace is released and the release.

Make sure you squirt your face before you let it go.

You can close your eyes. Release.

Eyes wide. Release.

The tension has gone. It is a state of complete relaxation. Breathe in and breathe out Feel peace and tranquility throughout your body.

It is now time for us to get to the next step.

Intensifying

The countdown technique is the most efficient method to take us into a deep state the trance state, also known as hypnosis. Simply count backwards from 10 20 or 100 or whatever number is right for you. You'll feel like you're sinking deeper and deeper each number.

It's normal for other ideas and thoughts to rise to the surface and appear to you as you go through the process. Just go through them and never stop in your count.

Suggestion

When you reach the conclusion of the state of deep relaxation the subconscious mind is open. Plan your suggestions by contemplating them before time. You're likely to be thinking about them right now, so now is the perfect moment to speak to yourself , and to make your subconscious aware of who you want to be and what you'd prefer to evolve.

Always refer to yourself with the pronoun of first person "I". Do not use phrases like "You can feel your bones growing longer".

Try thinking of something like "I am able to feel the entire cartilages and bones within my body getting longer" and "I can feel the growth hormones lengthening my bones as well as cartilages."

Visual suggestion is more efficient than semantic suggestion. It is all you need to do is imagine your bones stretching in a literal way or visualize your 4- inch taller self.

Be patient. The first results will be apparent within a couple of weeks. Otherwise you might need to look for other options.

Termination

Termination marks the line between hypnosis and conscious or between hypnosis and sleep. Even if you are able to fall asleep shortly after the end of your self-hypnosis however, you must locate a way to define the line since the two are totally distinct states.

For the second time counting is the most effective method to accomplish this. Make yourself promise yourself to awake and regain complete awareness once you count three. One two, three and then you're completely conscious. It's the end of your self-hypnosis exercise!

Chapter 8: Exercises To Get Taller

It is here that the real component of your program starts. If you believe that you're getting the correct kind of food and exercise, you must give your body some push to stimulate growth hormones.

The greatest thing of these workouts is the fact that they're fairly simple to perform. They're also simple to incorporate into your routine, without hassle in acquiring equipment or finding the ideal conditions.

The majority of the exercises you'll encounter will be the kind of stretching. This is due to the reason that increasing height is similar to stretching.

Bed Stretches

These are exercises that are able to do when you wake up. It is also possible to do them prior to bed However, dependent on your sleeping pattern The stretches may disrupt your sleep patterns.

The most basic bed stretch is to simply lie down in your bed and stretch your legs and arms as far as you are able to. After you have straightened your body out, turn around from one side of the bed to another.

After you're satisfied, raise your hips while lying on your the bed by lifting your body up using your hands. Your legs should be pointed straight upwards, while your head remains in the mattress. Do kicks as if you're moving in the air.

Stand up, and then move your chin toward your chest. Turn your head to the left and then to the right and then draw it backwards. Your neck should be being stretched.

Standing Stretches

Then, get up from your bed and stand up straight. Spread your arms out sideways and turn them around, creating small circles on your sides. Don't extend your elbows. You'll feel the movement through the shoulders. Be sure to turn to both sides.

In the beginning, assume the original position with your arms stretched out toward the sides. Now, twist your body to make one arm rise and the other goes down. Stretch towards your opposite end, then alternate. Do not extend your elbows, arms or neck.

Then, stand straight and extend both arms upwards. Be sure to place your ears within your arms. After that, stretch one arm and then the otherarm, trying to reach to the maximum distance you can to each side.

Extra Exercise Additional Exercise: Hanging. Look for a space within your home that has an aluminum horizontal bar that you can attach to. Hold the bar and allow your entire body to hang suspended in air. This is a great method of stretching. You can also try hanging onto something else, such as the door's ledge. Be careful, however you could result in accidents.

The training of your body to be More Taller

The next thing to improve will be your posture. It's the way you sit and position certain areas of your body whether you're walking, standing, and sitting. The effort you make into maintaining a good posture can make an enormous difference, particularly when you're getting older as one of the main reasons for height loss later in the course of.

A good posture practice doesn't only make you appear taller, but it actually makes you taller in the sense that it assists in the stretching exercises you're performing. Therefore, it's just as important as your stretching routine.

The posture issues are primarily focused on standing and sleeping postures as it's normal to be in a different position while sitting or walking. The practice of correct posture while in one position however, will help improve your posture throughout the day and positions.

Additionally one, but a person who has a good posture is likely to appear more attractive to the majority of people. They look more disciplined and friendly than those who's postures give others an impression that they have a low self-esteem or aren't social. The people who have a good posture are more likely to maintain concentration while working or listening to another person due to their better oxygenation and breathing.

Proper Sleeping Position

I've already discussed how to stretch when you wake up. Sleeping itself can be a way to stretch but it's more specifically, it involves the proper positioning of your body for the best sleep.

The majority of your growth and metabolism occurs while you're asleep and it's crucial to ensure that your body is in the best position for optimal growth. In reality, poor sleeping postures have been proven to be the reason for the deformation of your body over time and also severe body aches.

Take note of the below guidelines:

The reason sleeping promotes growth is that the person is in the position in which spinal discs aren't subjected to unwanted pressure. Any sleeping position that has an impact upon this principle is a bad (in in the sense it isn't suitable for height gain) posture for sleeping.

The ideal position for sleeping is to lie on the bed with your limbs in a relaxed position, and stretched. When you are in this position the entire body is free of tension which gives it the space to develop according to its own rate.

Don't lie on pillows, especially ones which are large. Contrary to popular opinion pillows can cause pain to the shoulder and neck area.

Imagine lying down in a position where you lay your head on the pillow . You'll think about how your neck is bent and how your shoulders curve. Compare these postures to the way you look standing up , and you'll be able to see how strange it feels. Beware of these positions that aren't natural.

* Ensure that you're getting enough rest. The amount of time required for a person varies from to the next, but the goal is always 8-10 hours of sleep per day. To aid you, think about studying the sleep cycle. It can help you determine the way your body sleeps and then wakes up in the most natural manner (as opposed to getting up feeling tired and stressed). In the opposite, you should ensure you don't go to bed with too many hours of sleep. This is not only unproductive It can also lead to fatigue, too.

Common Posture Problems

Proper posture goes beyond simply standing up straight, and trying to appear at the highest height you think you are. The truth is that posture is in the finer details, that is, in specific areas of your body, you may assume as correct posture is concerned.

Pelvis - Some people lean their pelvis to the side or outward. This can cause the body to move inward or outward and is not an ideal posture. If you're engaging in this without knowing it is important to be aware of the way you sit your pelvis when standing up. For this, you must get an accurate feel for your spine and stomach and determine if you feel tension on one side or the other. The most common rule of thumb is that your back and stomach muscles should not feel any pressure. If you're not, you're positioning your pelvis in the wrong way.

Many people are also in a position that is not correct due to a insufficient the back or stomach muscles. They can be fixed by using the stretching exercises described in the earlier chapter.

Shoulders - You'll be amazed by how many people knowingly are constantly slouching. Even those who believe they are sitting straight do slouch at times. It's commonplace nowadays when people use computers all day long, which means they tighten their shoulders not knowing that they are in an uncomfortable posture. A good ergonomics practice requires the shoulders to relax even when your hands are working.

People who write or type for long periods of time aren't expected to experience shoulder pain If they keep a good posture. Shoulders should be slanting downwards while in a comfortable position. This of course is in conjunction with sitting in the right kind of chair or when walking, wearing balanced kinds of bags (so that you don't press the back and shoulders in a dissimilar way).

Knock-Knees and Bowlegs People who exhibit these traits are obvious and may have already seen medical professionals, however in additional, there is a way to increase your chances by incorporating the exercise routines and diet recommended in this guide.

Be aware of your posture. We get used to the way we interact with people, particularly when we're relaxed that we slump, slouch or bend and place our bodies in uncomfortable positions. It's not until later that we regret the decision. It's a process that takes time, but soon it will become automatic to you.

79

Chapter 9: Which Actually Stunts Growth?

Understanding what drives growth is only half of the task. It is also crucial to understand what you can do to eliminate or fix the things that adversely affect growth rates. One of the main causes for the slowed growth of children is diseases and disorder. The most significant causes of this are lifestyle choicesthat can be criticized by any person who is committed to a disciplined lifestyle.

Physical disorders - Sometimes, people suffer from illnesses that impact their growth. Certain illnesses are genetic and others develop in different ways. They are treatable or prevented on a situation to individual basis. The most important thing to remember is that having a diagnosis of the conditions can help you know the extent to which you're at in terms of maximising the growth potential you have.

Osteoporosis causes an increase in calcium leading to bones being more prone to break. Calcium is essential to bone growth and overall growth. Hypothyroidism is a disorder that children are afflicted with, and it is also a factor in slowing growth. Hypogonadism, which decreases the body's estrogen levels as well as testosterone levels could cause growth issues during puberty.

There are a variety of disorders or diseases and deformities that can affect the growth of children. The main thing to remember from all of this is that parents must treat them as quickly as they can, particularly when they first appear in childhood.

Unsafe Weight Lifting - Logically weight lifting is a stumbling block to the growth of a person since they make your body sink, working with gravity for so long. It's not the way it works however.

The fact is that correct weight training can encourage growth since, as a method of bodybuilding it permits you to increase the strength and flexibility in your physique. What hinders growth is ineffective weight lifting that usually creates bad posture and muscles strain.

When you exercise, make certain to follow the guidelines of your trainers to ensure that you exercise correctly and at the correct speed. This will not only aid in your growth and stronger, but it can also help prevent injuries too.

Smoking is a major cause of smoking cigarettes to stunted growth. The reason behind this is that smoking decreases blood circulation and oxygen which is crucial for growth.

If you're determined to increase your the height you desire, it might be beneficial to quit smoking cigarettes. It's essential to have to have a better body.

In the event that a whole chapter was focused on proper nutrition to ensure optimal growth, it's a matter of saying that people who are malnourished tend to be less efficient in their growth. However, it is not enough how crucial it is for one to eat three squares daily and to avoid eating junk food for an overall better life style. A lot of children nowadays are malnourished as a result an unhealthy diet. As an adult it is your top priority to make sure that your children eat a balanced diet.

Chapter 10: Additional Strategies To Control Height

There are many other methods to appear taller, in addition to being physically larger. Although they may not be the only solution to height issues, it can be a big difference in the effort to create an impression.

How to Make Yourself Seem More Taller

You'll be shocked by the amount of famous or people you've met who appear more taller than they actually are. They employ subtle techniques to give the illusion. Here are some simple tricks you can try at home:

Shoes - It's not difficult for women to wear heels however the reality that heels are noticeable can dispel the notion of being more tall. It's just that you appear to be an inch shorter when you wear heels. The secret lies in the Insoles and shoes which are made to make you appear larger. Insoles and shoes can be purchased in many shops, and they can also be customized. They can add up to 1 inch to your height.

Clothing - Just as wearing large clothes makes you appear smaller, but wearing the right type of clothes will make you appear larger as well. Although dark solids and vertical lines are thought of as more slimming in appearance, these actually provide an elongating effect too. Consider wearing clothes in only one color that runs from the top to the bottom and you'll notice how taller you'll appear. Avoid oversized clothes or smaller sizes because they make your appearance appear less attractive. Remember you're trying to appear taller, not awkward.

Hair - Do not wear long, hair that is not covered, as it tends to cover your neck and make it appear that you're taller than you actually are. There are a variety of hairstyles that increase your overall height by giving your hair volume. This is the simplest way for men to increase some inches. The professionals working in salons are knowledgeable about how to style hair which affects how the height of a person is perceived.

Techniques to avoid

This article is about ways to make yourself more imposing. When we say "natural" we refer to anything that's not ordeal nor can it be risky to risk permanent damage to your body. Many people go to such measures to alter their appearance which can end up harming more than they help themselves.

Naturally, the only thing you should avoid is having surgical procedures. The people who advocate for natural methods of living a healthy lifestyle consider that surgery are only used when they are absolutely required. They shouldn't be viewed as an alternative to any kind. Apart from the fact that they're dangerous, procedures can be extremely expensive and difficult to manage considering that there are more affordable and more secure alternatives, and surgeries don't make much difference.

There are other types of medications that are designed to boost the human growth hormone, or HGH supply. This is a great option for people who want to boost the amount of HGH in their bodies however, it's not something you should consider in the hopes of getting larger. While a lack of HGH during childhood may impede growth, taking too much of it because of supplementing even when you aren't required can be harmful to your body too.

If you are feeling that you need to consider surgery (e.g. in the case of one leg being shorter than the other one and it causes a change in posture and creates discomfort) or you are taking HGH supplements and make it a priority to speak with your physician. They'll be able to determine if you are able to undergo these procedures safely and may even recommend more alternatives that aren't harmful so you don't need to undergo the arduous procedures.

Chapter 11: Genes And You

Before we can discuss more about natural ways to increase our height, we need to examine the genetics, gene recombination and the way that these factors affect the height of a person.

The term "Genes" was derived from the Greek term" genos" which means "race which is also known as offspring". Genes are distinct DNA molecules that alter traits that are passed down through generations. This discovery about Genes resulted from an Gregorian monk's simple test of inheritance. This led to the conclusion that parents' characteristics are passed on to their children.

The traits of height unlike other traits that are common are thought to be extremely difficult to grasp or even anticipate, particularly when there is genetic recombination. Genetic recombination refers specifically to genes that have no traits from the parents, which means that the genes have merged the characteristics of the parents, so and that no distinct characteristic of the parents can be evident in the children. For instance the combination of a short and a tall one could lead in a child who is average height.

The definition of an ethnicity by sociology, is defined by cultural similarities as well as cultural variations. An ethnic group can comprise blood-related humans or those who adhere to the same set of rules. Certain researchers have predicted that in ethnic groups, the likelihood of a person mating with someone else within the same ethnic group is extremely high. Because of this repeated event researchers believe that regardless of how large the cultural group might be, it has the potential of being blood relatives. This has led to patterns on the various characteristics a particular group is known to have.

The belief was that patterns of growth differ across various ethnic groups. There is a belief that subsequent generations of different ethnic groups are not just determined by blood type of the generation before them as well as the ways of life practiced by ancestral ancestors.

In support of these claims as per research findings conducted by researchers, those from the African-Caribbean areas are larger and heavier than those from the African-Caribbean regions, while Asian as well as Chinese groups are smaller and lighter than Caucasians (white people of European descent). Recently, a research group disproved this idea and suggested that being born in the population could mean an increased chance that you will be taller than if you live in a different location with different norms. The difference is that African-Caribbean communities are famous for their shipwork and manpower. They have been known to complete things with their hands, for example, transporting things in groups or simply completing tasks with their hands. Since these activities are carried out repeatedly, kids in this category have a good probability of inheriting the genes from their fathers.

A Direct Connection

The genes that determine height are part of our DNA. Studies have revealed that around 75 percent of our height is derived from the blueprint of our lives (DNA) and the remaining 25% are affected by external factorslike routine actions and positive surroundings. Studies have shown that about 80% of the people within a particular population have a height determined by genes and that other 20% were able to attain their height because of their surroundings. Thus, it can be said that your height doesn't solely depend on genetics. Another interesting fact concerning genes is that scientists are currently researching accurate predictions of the height of offsprings.

Growing in height naturally can be difficult for some. Genetics can be difficult to change , however, If we are able to do our best and work hard and persevere, we'll surely reach our ideal height. In the subsequent chapters, factors that impact the height of people living in different cultures, with different beliefs, and pursuing different ways of life will be examined. Alongside the factors that affect height are the natural strategies we propose that can be easily appropriate to anyone who wants to be taller but not spending all of their time.

Diet and Its Effect

One thing that could raise the height of your body naturally can be your diet, because consuming more nutrients in the process of digestion and bone growth will definitely benefit. China often advised its citizens to consume food that was healthier. This led to the height average in China was increased by about six inches. While other countries that aren't eating enough nutritious food, or are suffering from malnutrition, have smaller people.

A diet or meal plan is the arrangement of the consumed food, the types of food items to be consumed, as well as the timing at which food that is cooked will be consumed. A diet plan could be developed every day, weekly or monthly, and even every year. Many people make meal plans in order to keep the healthiest diet possible or to meet certain objectives or goals. For the diet plan or meal strategy to be successful it is necessary to first study the body. It is essential to understand the way your body functions to ensure that you can adhere to a plan of eating that's suitable for your specific needs. It is best if you discuss this with the help of a dietician (an specialist in human nutrition).

Nowadays, many people prefer to search on online on the World Wide Web for meal plans, rather than going to a clinic for a consultation with the doctor personally. The majority of the plans available on the internet are based on different food groups. Food groups are defined as foods that share biological resemblances. There are five main food groups, including the dairy group and the fruit group, grains as well as the lean meats, eggs, fish, poultry tofu, tofu, nuts and seeds group, and finally the legumes, vegetables and beans group.

Focusing on what's important

Within the dairy group there are dairy products that are high in calcium. Calcium is crucial for anyone to maintain healthy and strong bones. The majority of foods belonging to different groups don't have as much calcium as those belonging to the dairy category. Fruits are the group where we can find food items that are high in minerals, vitamins, as well as other nutrients that aid in the development and growth within the organism.

The grains are also referred to in"the "cereal category" as well as the "carbohydrates group" is the foods that are high in carbohydrates. Certain foods in this group could be very high in fat, sugar and sodium.

This fourth category, which is also called"lean meats and poultry, eggs, tofu, nuts and seeds group "lean meats and fish, poultry eggs, tofu nuts as well as seeds" is where you will find food items that are high of protein. Protein is crucial for height growth. The legumes, vegetables, as well as beans category is in which we can also find food items high in minerals, vitamins as well as other nutrients that are essential for the growth of the body.

There are plenty of foods that are rich in minerals and vitamins required to grow, such as fish and milk (both fish and milk are part of the category of "grow food group" which is a category of food with a high protein levels) and both are rich in calcium, the primary ingredient in the construction of bones. Insufficient intake of calcium can lead in Osteoporosis as well as Calcium Deficiency (hypocalcaemia). Fish and Milk are high in Vitamin D which can improve Calcium absorption by bones. Vitamin D is involved in balancing hormones , too. Insufficient levels of this Vitamin could cause the development of rickets (disease of having weak bone or weak ones) and bone deformities. Fish and milk are also high of Vitamin B12 or the so-called Riboflavin, which is known to stimulate the development of bones.

Spinach is a nutritious food that is that is rich in vitamins and minerals particularly those that influence the height. Magnesium is one of them. It aids in maintaining the density of bones (the bone strength) by directing calcium toward the bones. The absence of Magnesium is the cause of Hypocalcaemia. Spinach also contains Potassium that causes the body to become more acidic. The body must avoid becoming acidic, and if it is, it will be able to signal your bones to break down components of it to help balance the acid base levels.

Phosphorus can also be found in Spinach It is also well-known for its role in maintaining bone health. Furthermore, Spinach contains many proteins that help keep the bone structure in good shape. This particular type of food also contains Vitamin A that is needed for the production of protein.

Chocolate oysters, peas and apricots contain Zinc and is essential to maintaining bone health. Children who do not have sufficient Zinc is more likely to be of low or less-than-average height.

Pork and rice are significant food sources for Vitamin B1 that is essential to promote growth and healthy digestion. As you can see, many of the minerals and vitamins are important to aid in bone health. This is due to the fact that bone growth is closely linked to the height. Be aware that maintaining your bones in good health is about increasing your height.

We should not only be aware of the food we consume and how much water we consume every day. Research suggests that on an average humans should be capable of drinking six to eight glasses of fluid. Drinking water does more than provide our body with nutrients but also enhances the benefits of minerals, vitamins and other nutrients are consumed to gain height.

A Critical Reminder

If you are reading this you're likely to be thinking about filling your fridge with food items described in the chapter. You may be thinking of exclusively rely on them as food. It's not a good choice. Make sure that your diet regimen is in line with what experts advise. This will assist you in choosing which meal to have in the future, and also aid in determining your food intake. Make sure to incorporate the food items included in this list into well-portioned meals that are nutritionally balanced schedules.

Benefits of Activities

It is also possible to naturally increase your height without the need of extravagant. The activities that help increase your height are related with stretching the bones in the greatest way particularly your vertebra once they've fully developed. Methods to correct how you posture yourself and stretching muscles vertically could help to increase your height.

The most well-known exercise to increase your height gradually is stretching. It involves flexing the muscle's growth points to allow the growth. The term "stretching" can be divided into seven kinds, namely:

* Ballistic

* Isometric

* PNF (Proprioceptive Neuromuscular Facilitation)

* Dynamic

* Active

* Passive

* Static

Note you must be aware that Ballistic, Isometric, and PNF stretching rely on the body's motion, causing you to test your limits in terms of speed and endurance. The three stretches mentioned are are not advised and must be avoided by everyone who wants to increase their height. They're also too long for those who are growing their bones, for instance teens and children. Why? It's mostly because of their more flexible than normal in bones and joints which means that stretching for long periods of time can cause damage to connective tissue.

However, dynamic stretches consist of controlled leg and arm swing movements, which are more gentle in comparison to Ballistic stretching. Active stretching involves maintaining a stretched place for as long as the maximum amount of time you are able to such as keeping your leg straight for 30 minutes or longer. Active stretching is completed without assistance while passive stretching requires equipment or support from a person or object. For instance, doing breaks on the ground will help to maintain your extended posture. The floor acts as an apparatus during this moment. When you are able to hold your knee using your hand, your hand acts as the apparatus.

Static and passive stretching is very similar. Only difference between them is static stretching is stretching to the maximum extent, but it doesn't require the use of an apparatus or require any movements.

Stretching in basic ways like sit and reach or bridge stretch can be a great way to get the job done. However, in order to reap the most benefit from stretching, it is essential to perform stretching for every 15 minutes or so throughout the each day. Another method to stretch your spine and joints is to keep them upside down. This way, you'll challenge gravity (which can hinder us from increase our height and forces the body down). You can perform this feat using an exercise bar, or anything which can raise your weight off the ground. Repeat it continuously for an increase in your height.

There are a lot of ways to boost your height, like jumping rope. It doesn't just help you slim down, but it can also help the calf muscles extend vertically. Additionally, skipping causes muscle to expand and contract (especially the ligaments and tendons) which makes their muscles more flexible. Skipping rope can also assist in the process of elongating your bones. Additionally the fact that when you jump rope, you'll be higher, which helps in decompressing your spine and correcting posture.

Power of Slumber

Typically, doctors and other health experts would suggest an evening of restful sleep to ensure better health. This is accepted as fact since the right amount of sleep can also aid in the growth of humans. Researchers have found that during the night, your height gets modified as your backbone relaxes, and expands slightly. In addition, eight hours of rest is sufficient time for your body to heal and allow your brain to rest and slow down. This means that the pituitary gland works to release growth hormone. Thus, the longer you are asleep, the greater the likelihood that growth hormones will be released by your body.

It is to be expected that the lack of sleep can result in a slowdown in growth due to absence of growth hormone.

Swimming Solution

Health experts have also pointed that swimming is among of the best sports to improve your height as it involves both your feet and hands working simultaneously. The most effective way to increase your height is believed to be the"breaststroke that requires you to move from your sides to the breast in all lengths in both directions , and you feet are required to paddle in a single direction. This will result in stretching your muscles and spine. Furthermore, it assists in encouraging your body's production of hormones like growth because swimming increases both of the key elements required for the secretion of growth hormones including lactate and Nitric oxide. Studies have also shown that children who regularly swim tend to become larger than those who do not swim.

You might want to think about doing Yoga

Another beneficial way to increase your height is Yoga. While it doesn't aid in the growth of bones however, it can help in stretching your spine and improving your posture and spinal endurance. A few of the techniques utilized in Yoga that can assist you in growing taller are ones like Ardha yoga poses, Kurmasana, and Bhujangasana.

Ardha Kurmasana is also referred to for its "half tortoise posture". It's done by bent knees on the floor, and then arching your back toward your knees. This will ensure that your knees and your chest remain close to one the other as you raise your arms out in front while keeping both hands closed with your palms facing one another. This pose should resemble the tortoise when done. This position helps you prevent the pain of your back and spinal problems. In addition, it helps lengthen your spine.

Bhujangasana also often referred to as "snake posture" is achieved by placing your feet on the floor and lifting your head and torso up before bending your back slightly leaving both feet down on the floor. Bhujangasana improves spine flexibility length, strength, and flexibility.

Think about Pilates

Pilates is among the most well-known and extensive core exercisesthat aid in increasing growth as does Yoga. It doesn't aid in boosting the size of bones however it can help in extending the backbone. Pilate is a series of exercises that are primarily designed to build the core (referring to muscles that run between your back and the abdominal) strength. One of the routines in Pilates is called the Pilates Hundreds. It is performed with knees bent while making sure your feet are on the floor as you stretch your shoulders and head while keeping the lower back that is still press down on the floor. You will then need to position your arms to the sides of your hip and slowly push them upwards and downwards. This assists in strengthening your spine and also in increasing the endurance of your spine.

What to Avoid

To get positive results, it is best to be careful about certain actions. Things like smoking can harm the cells that allow growth hormones be released. It is also advised to stay clear of drinking alcohol in large quantities. A lot of alcohol can damage the liver. In addition smoking can harm the liver too. The liver plays an essential part in the creation of proteins, which are required by bones. Without it, maintaining the bone's structure is difficult.

One of the things you should be aware of when trying to increase your height is to do extensive training and weight lifting as they can cause confusion to your body and cause it to focus on building muscle. However, growing your height will require light exercise to relax and stretch your backbone and maintain a healthy posture. When a person is stressed, they are susceptible to producing negative hormones, which can adversely affect your body's various cycles. Therefore, the reduction of stress is recommended as it will not only aid in the direction of your vertebra, but it also aids in maintaining an efficient production of Human Growth Hormone.

The Role of Environment

The environment that the person is living in may impact the height. If we look closely those who live in urban regions tend to be more taller than those living in rural regions.

Additionally, some researchers claim that the socio-economic standing of a person greatly influences the chance of increasing height via natural methods, but certain researchers disagree. The only requirement is to be ingenious enough to seek out alternatives when resources aren't there.

Humans have built communities and prospered around the availability of potable, clean fresh air and water from the beginning of time. It is essential for our survival and development. Air pollution can severely impact our health and alter the body's systems, which could slow the growth. Nearly everything that is an outgrowth of our culture can be found in our drinking water as well as the surrounding air. Consuming unclean and polluted water could cause serious damage to the digestive tract. Infectious diseases can transferred through contaminated water or from the filthy air. Airborne and waterborne diseases can have significant effects on the height of the person.

The question now is how can we grow in height while living in areas that are polluted? It is just a matter of being careful.

Drinking clean water can aid in the absorption of minerals and vitamins can have more effect on the body. You must ensure that you are clean when preparing food to safeguard our immune system and to prevent illnesses that could affect our health. This is due to diseases that reduce the body's capacity to grow. Keep in mind that a secure and healthy environment, as well as living a healthy life style, improves the likelihood of growing in height.

Being in a healthy environment can significantly impact your height since, in part your height is influenced by the surroundings you live in. The surroundings can trigger factors that can greatly affect your height. A setting that allows you to perform activities that increase your height with no disturbance, or a space in which you can do yoga in peace, will increase your chance of growing more taller.

Also, a clean environment can assist in making your brain feel relaxed so that your pituitary gland will perform more efficiently. An alcohol-free and smoke-free environment can also be of great assistance, particularly when it comes to preventing the growth deficiencies. In addition having the ideal conditions for sleeping is essential for anyone who wants to grow their height because of the importance of sleeping without disturbance when growing. A place in which you have access to food high in minerals and vitamins that are essential for growth will allow you to strengthen your bones and muscles.

Learn from History

It is believed that the Nilotic People (Indigenous people who mainly reside in Southern Sudan) are described as having legs that are long and slim bodies that make them appear tall. The distinctive features mentioned above are further explained by scientists as a characteristic that these people have because of the need to be able to cope with hot temperatures.

Nilotic people are further divided into a variety of groups. Two of them are Shilluk and Dinka in which their average size of people from Shilluk who were measured of 5'11 inches. The average height of people of Dinka which was recorded was 6 feet. It was before wars started to get underway. After the wars, the refugees were measured once more which led to the change in their height. Their average is at present 5 feet and 7 inches. One possible explanation is that war prevented the refugees from receiving enough food and rest.

In addition to the Nilotic people , the children of Guatemala also have shown the sudden shift. This was noted by Barry Bogin who conducted his research in the early 1970s. He noted their height and average. In the Guatemalan Civil war, the Guatemala Maya children fled to the United States of America. Following this war ended, they took measurements of the height of children aged between 6 and 12 and observed that the measurements were higher than those recorded before the war started. This is because the people who were refugees could get adequate nutrition, and in a setting that allowed their development.

The two studies mentioned above demonstrate that the environment has the ability to alter the height of the earth and keep it in place or alter it. This was evident in both instances. Thus, the environmental environments and the individual's growth are closely linked. In terms of their importance to you, in addition to being a reminder to remain in a setting that promotes the growth of your body, it is important to be aware of the places which could actually hinder the development of your body You must get away from environments that where you are constantly stressed and significantly.

Chapter 12: Actors Subject To Growth

Nutrition

Absolutely the quality, quantity and kind of food we consume can affect your height and growth and overall health. We can't stress enough the significance of what you eat determines the amount of growth you could achieve. The type of food you consume will either increase or hinder your growth.

After careful consideration and investigation the daily amount of carbohydrates, protein and fats, as well as water can be reached if the following items are consumed regularly. Be aware that this is only a suggestion and you're at liberty to explore your own ideas. Eat rationally to boost your height, have lots of vitality and lead an active and fulfilling life.

Food Patterns

Take a minimum of two hours prior to starting your workout. It's a known truth that the levels of insulin rise immediately following a large, food intake. Insulin reduces HGH release, and a large meal drains blood of your muscle and directs it to your stomach. It is important to eat right after exercising. crucial to ensure that muscle dystrophy does not be a problem.

Food intake prior to exercise

Any carbohydrate, such as bread, baked potato, jam spaghetti, cereal, or even cereals are excellent options. Make sure to consume foods that have moderate glycemic index, to ensure that your body will always have an ongoing supply of energy during exercise.

Eating after exercise

We suggest one cup of orange juice, mixed with a cup of water, following an excellent

training or exercising. Be careful not to drink right after having exercised for long or fast times as you could choke. Let your breath stabilise before drinking. For foods, anything that is high in protein is an excellent source, paired with a little carbohydrates. A optimal proportion is 1/2 protein, 3/4 carbohydrate.Mixing an instant breakfast of 1 cup milk, and a small banana is an excellent combination. Don't mix hot water with protein because it could deform on an molecular level and reduce its effectiveness.

What should you be aware of to

Don't eat your food in large amounts. It is advised to eat five to seven meals per day. Be sure to avoid eating for at least the two hours before you go to bed. Consuming food prior to bedtime blocks HGH release, and your efforts will be wasted. Foods with high levels of saturated fats, rich in sugar and processed food are best avoided. Avoid drinking excessive amounts of milk or water at a moment. Drink water at regular intervals (approx. eight glasses of fluid per day).

Useful proteins

The ones that are readily digested in the blood stream are the most beneficial. Examples of these proteins are milk, whey protein cheese, yoghurt and even boiled chicken. Proteins such as meat and eggs are difficult for your body to absorb and require longer to pass through the digestive system.

Fibre

The consumption of extra protein isn't natural. But for the purposes of this article, we need plenty of protein. To ensure that you don't become constipated, take a bite of cucumbers or "boiled" carrots along with your meals. They are a great source of fiber, so you'll be regular and avoid stomach cramps.

Food to grow

Your bones require phosphorus magnesium, and calcium while your muscles require protein, water and

carbohydrates to increase. Because you're growing bigger, your bones and muscles are growing longer and bigger. Consider what foods to eat , and the best time to eat it, then let your common sense become your guide.

The ideal diet that you must follow to increase your height is one that has a balanced mix of vitamins, proteins and minerals. Your diet must include the three types of nutrition such as protein, carbohydrate and Fats.

Carbohydrate

A common diet that slows growth in height is one that is high in carbs.

Carbohydrates typically contain things like bread, rice potato, corn, potatoes and many other cereal grains. Beware of eating too many carbs as they provide lots of energy (calories) but they lack important nutrients that aid your body in its growth.

This is why Asian people are smaller than people of European as well as American people. Asian individuals' diets are predominantly comprised of carbs-based food items like corn or rice however, European and American consumers consume more protein-rich meals. Therefore, don't consume bread, rice, potatoes or cereal grains your primary foods if are looking to increase your height!

Fats

Another diet that is known to hinder growing tall is one that has excessive amounts of fats (fats). There are two types of fats, saturated as well as unsaturated fats. saturated fats are generally bad because they contain high levels of cholesterol. They could cause heart diseases because the arteries can be blocked by fat material. In addition, saturated fats are loaded with a significant amounts of calories which could easily add to the weight you carry. The weight gain is a threat to height because the more weight you carry the smaller you appear. Avoid eating too much saturated fats.

Animal products such as pork, chicken and beef are rich of saturated fats. Therefore, you should be careful not to eat excessive amounts of them. Unsaturated fats are better since they are a lesser quantity of calories and cholesterol. Because you need fats to help insulate your body and control your metabolism, it is better take in more unsaturated fats to fulfill the body's demands.

Vegetable oils contain a large quantity of fats that are unsaturated. The most commonly used vegetable oils that are unsaturated include corn, soy cottonseed, cottonseed and safflower oils. Take note that raw milk as well as butter are full of saturated fats. Therefore, you should drink milk that is skimmed and cook using the vegetable oil instead. Desserts like cookies cakes, ice cream, and cake are also very rich in of calories and saturated fats, and you should avoid eating too much of them.

Protein

To grow larger, your body needs minerals, vitamins, and proteins more frequently than fats, carbohydrates and carbohydrates. Proteins are comprised of some or all groups of amino acid chains. They are the primary constituents of all living cells . They comprise a myriad of compounds including hormones, enzymes, and antibodies, that are essential to function properly in an organism. They are vital to our diet as animals to aid in the development and repair of tissue , and consequently, it is important to consume a significant amounts of protein if you wish to increase your height. The most nutritious food sources that provide complete protein (those which have the highest amount of amino acids necessary for growth) include eggs, fish milk, legumes, and eggs. These are the most abundant all 20 amino acids and include the eight vital amino acids which can't be made by our bodies. So, you can replace bread, rice and hamburgers with eggs, fish as well as skim milk.

These are natural resources of some amino acids.

Amino Acids Natural Sources Function

Arginine Brown Rice

Carob

Chocolate

Nuts

Oatmeal

Popcorn

Raisins

Raw cereals

Sesame seeds

Sunflower seeds

Whole-wheat flour products function as a protein building blocks for all proteins.

Human growth hormone is stimulated

L-Lysine Cheese

Eggs

Fish

Lima beans

Milk

Potatoes

Red meat

Soy products

The role of yeast is to be an vital building block of all proteins

Promotes growth,tissue repair and production of antibodies,hormones,enzyms

Tyrosine Almonds

Avocados

Bananas

Cheese

Cottage cheese

Lima beans

Non-fat dried milk

Peanuts

Herrings that have been prickled

Pumpkin seeds

Sesane seeds are a key protein building blocks for all proteins

Can induce significant short-term increases of blood levels of norepinephrine,dopamine and epinephirine.May be harmful at times and helpful at others.Don't take without medical supervision.

Amino Acids Natural Sources Function

Taurine Eggs

Fish

Meat

Milk could be beneficial in the treatment of epilepsy.

It is a building block that can be used to construct all proteins.

Controls the nervous system

L-Carnitine Avocados

Dairy products

Lamb, red meats and beef

Tempeh (fermented soybean product) Helps to promote healthy growth as well as development

Folic Acid Barley

Beans

Brewer's yeast

Calves liver

Endive Fruits

Garbanzo beans(chick peas)

Green leafy

Vegetables

Lentils

Orange juice

Oranges

Peas

Rice helps promote the normal process of red blood cell production

Maintains the nervous system, intestinal tract, sex organs, white blood cells, normal patterns of growth.

Regulates development of the embryo and fetal stage

Alcohol, Tobacco , and other drugs

Do not waste your money or your health with smoking cigarettes, alcohol, or drugs. Spend your money on healthy food items or high-quality supplements. Learn how to say "NO to:

* self destructive drugs

* alcohol that is intoxicating

* cigarettes that can be poisonous

Make sure you choose healthy with natural and organic products that offer health, energy endurance, energy and general wellbeing.

Tips for healthy eating

1. Eat regularly during the day.

2. Do not skip meals.

3. Do not forget to take a breakfast. Start your day with a an adequate and balanced meal.

4. Make sure to taste and chew your food thoroughly.

5. Variate your menu.

6. Beware of sweets, pastries crisps, soda drinks, sweets or anything with only a small or zero nutritional worth.

7. Beware of your salt intake. It may cause hypertension.

8. Take a large amount of fresh vegetables and raw juice. Select whole wheat bread.

9. Consume at least six (6) or eight (8) glasses of vegetable juice or water or juices that are sugar-free per day.

10.You must also consume milk.

11.Eat nutritious food supplements of good quality daily.

12.After every meal, you must have a rest. Do not start exercise or work immediately following.

Vitamins and Minerals

A sufficient and adequate supply of minerals and vitamins should be consumed to allow all biological functions of the body including development and growth to function in the best possible way. Consuming fish is of the utmost importance because it contains a lot of minerals other foods do not have, and can help your body to grow. Certainly, minerals and vitamins are essential for bone size and density. The most crucial mineral to consider is calcium. Be aware that popular drinks and foods may cause calcium inhibition and slow growth. These calcium inhibitors include soft drinks, coffee, that contain refined sugar, a concentrated sweetener, excessive salt, high fats as well as alcohol and cigarettes. Limit or eliminate the consumption of these food items as well drinks, if you are looking to get taller.Therefore the most appropriate diet to get taller must consist of protein-rich food items like fish, meat that is not saturated eggs, milk and legumes. They are also vitamin-rich food items like vegetables, fruits, and animal livers; minerals-rich food like milk, seafood and dairy products.

Sleep

Sleep is the time of day that your mind has entrusted to heal, remove as well as replenish the body. It can also control your body's ability to expand. So, it is sensible to ensure you are in the right sleeping environment so that you can benefit the growth-enhancing rewards.You might be shocked to find out that we're larger when we wake up than at night. Because of gravity's law that our bodies, when in a sitting position are drawn towards the ground. When we reach the time we finish your day discs in the spine are compressed by weight of our bodies. At night the spinal column remains lying in a relaxed and stretched out position. Be aware of this and make use of the time to stretch in a proper way. Get up at six, lunch at 10 and dinner at 6 and bed at 10. will make man live 10 times. The need to sleep is part of all human beings. It is a necessity for us to live. Sleep deprivation for adults or children could have serious consequences.

Sleep is essential.

Sleep is thought to be the most affordable medication. People who are stressed or suffering from illness require sound sleep over all other things. Most of the time, there is no better way to fight illness than a night of rest. Sleep increases your energy levels It also boosts the energy levels of your central nervous system.

It soothes cartilage, bones and the muscle tissues. It eliminates fatigue from your body when you sleeping. Toxins get eliminated through the pores of your skin. Therefore, it is imperative to take an energizing shower in the morning. An energetic person is able to work to their fullest potential and last longer. A well-rested person also appears more attractive and radiant.

Tips to get taller while sleeping

It is during sleep that growth hormone can do its job of enhancing the thickness and increasing the length of your bones. Therefore, a proper amount of sleep (not longer, but the more) and a proper sleeping position is crucial for your body's growth. Sleep is defined as a period of rest for body and mind that occurs when eyes shut and consciousness is totally or only partially lost, meaning you experience a decline in body movement and sensitivity in response to stimuli external.

While you sleep deeply, growth hormone that is produced by your pituitary gland gets released into the blood stream and is absorbed by your body, causing growth and lengthening of bones. So, it is important to get "deep levels of" sleep on a regular basis to be able to coordinate your workouts and the right diet. Below are some suggestions on how to get to a deep sleep.

* Rest on a comfortable but firm bed. If the mattress isn't enough, put a piece of plywood on top of the mattress. If you sleep on a firm surface,

it will help align your spine into the normal position. This can lengthen your spine and allow the growth hormone to flow easily throughout the body.

* Make sure you sleep in a space which is quiet, dark and clean. Avoid exposure to bright light when you sleep. The light will cause your brain to remain awake.

* It is essential to sleep in a air-conditioned room. Do not be scared to open the windows especially in the winter. It's better to lay on a blanket of extra wool instead of breathing in polluted air. The quality of oxygen-rich air you breathe has an impact on the growth of your body. Air quality issues can hinder your body from growing while you sleep.

Make sure you sleep in soft, clean and comfortable clothing. Uncomfortable clothing can hinder circulation of blood and cause you to change positions several times throughout the night, which can prevent your body from falling asleep. Be aware that growth hormones can only be effective once you are in deep sleep.

Make sure to keep your feet and hands warm. Studies have proven that warm feet and hands aid in triggering REM (rapid eye movements) deeper sleep. Cold feet and hands will prevent you from falling asleep.

Drink a large glass of water prior to going to bed and after you awake, this will help cleanse your system. Milk is also a great way to help you to sleep. It is a source of amino acid known as tryptophan. It is responsible for the effects of an serotonin. Avoid eating any food or drinks which contain nicotine, caffeine or alcohol for at least 5 to 4 hours prior to going to go to bed. Nicotine and caffeine can be stimulants that prevent you from falling asleep. Avoid eating having a big food intake within 3 to 4 hours prior your bedtime.

Exercise during the day to aid in sleeping better in the evening.

• A bath prior to bed. This can help you sleep better because it cleanses your body and relaxes tension muscles.

* Relax completely as well as deep breaths for several moments before going to the bed.

Relax from head to foot. Shut your eyes to ease each part of your body. Complete breathing exercises by using the three steps: (1) Inhale slowly and deeply through your nose for 3 to 5 second to ensure that your stomach is also expanding the chest muscles expand. (2) Continue to hold your breath for 3 - 5 minutes, then tighten the stomach muscles slowly. (3) Inhale slowly and deeply through the nose and mouth. This breathing exercise can assist in smoothing your blood circulation and prepare your body for rest.

Keep a routine of sleeping in the same way every day and on weekends. This will allow you to establish a routine of sleep. Your brain sends you "sleep signal" approximately at the same time each day, which helps you sleep faster and easier.

Every person has their particular daily needs for sleep. There is no truth to the statement that the more time you spend sleeping the better to grow. Insufficient sleep can make your body develop inactivity and slow your metabolism, which increases the chance of you gaining weight. A typical young adult growing in age needs minimum 8 hours of of sleep each day. Teens require at least 9 hours of sleep. This is an average and might not be the case for you.

The most effective way to determine the precise amount of sleep you require is to not estimate it anyhow. Simply sleep in the early hours every evening. Avoid using any alarm clock and then let yourself get up on your own. Your body is a biological clock, which can decide the amount of sleep it requires. If you maintain a regular sleep habits and don't break it (by making yourself stay up late or wake up early) your body will take take care of itself.

* It's also easy to determine the amount of sleep you've had every day. If you feel alert and do not feel tired or sleepy throughout the day You probably got enough rest the night before. If not, it is time to adjust your schedule and attempt to rest longer.

The correct posture to sleep is essential to your growth in the night. Correct posture during sleep will help stretch your spine as well as increase your height. Sleeping in poor posture could put pressure on your shoulders, neck and back, and slow your growth while you sleep.

You should sleep on your back and rest an elongated pillow between your knees. This will help align your spine correctly and help prevent any backaches that result from lying in a bent posture. Moving your feet and knees slightly can help your brain receive more oxygen-rich blood.

The more oxygen that your brain receives, the greater the amount of amount of energy you'll have to boost your growth while you sleep.

* Lay on your side by bending your knees. This can help flatten the back. A pillow that is flat can be utilized to help support the neck, particularly in cases where shoulders are wide.

Don't use a high pillows. If you are lying on your back, with the head resting upon a pillow that is high your neck may be bent inwards, and your back is positioned in an unnatural way. This can cause strain to your neck, shoulders and back. It can also hinder growth because your spine is in a slouche for most in the night. Avoid sleeping with your head down. This can increase swayback and stress shoulders and neck.

* "Early to bed, then early to rise, helps to make a man well-nourished, wealthy and smart". Keep in tune with nature. The more we separate ourselves from nature, the more likely we are unsatisfied and disengaged with ourselves.

Appearance

Through cleverly organizing your visual components of clothing and their appearance by cleverly arranging the visual elements of clothes, you can alter how your body is perceived , making you appear larger. To overcome your height-related disadvantages during an interview for a job or on for a romantic rendezvous, use these guidelines:

Hair style

Get the hairstyle that creates the illusion of being more taller. To make you appear taller, a hairstyle should be thin on the sides and taller in the top. This could create the illusion of as big as an inch higher. Don't have a wide hairstyle. Also, a head that is bald can make a person appear smaller.

Beware of clothes that have horizontal lines. Belts are vertical, so be sure to hide it under your clothing.

.Avoid clothing with a tartan or checkered pattern. Beware of cuffs that can make your legs appear smaller.

* Dress in clothes that have horizontal lines or striping. Stripping or vertical lines can make one appear slimmer, and thinness gives the appearance of greater height.

Don't wear sharply contrasted clothes and pants which will reveal the leg length, making your appearance appear smaller.

* Dress in clothes that have shoulder pads. Shoulder pads can make your shoulders appear larger and make your body appear slimmer.

• Wear shoes that make you appear larger. If you're a woman you should have no problem doing this as you will be able to find many female footwear with two or three inches of heels. For men, choose shoes that have thick soles to give the appearance of the height.

Beware of clothes composed of bulky and heavy fabric. They increase width and, consequently, reduce the visual impact.

* Wear cuffless pants in order to give your legs a longer look.

* Dress in the right coat or jacket, which is the right length. They should be finished at the point where the buttocks join the legs.

Color

• Match the color of your pants with your shoes ' colour to make your legs appear longer.

The lengthening of your upper body by wearing an appropriate belt to match your top.

* Dark hues like navy blue, black and charcoal grey show strength and competence. More light-colored shades can make you appear more relaxed. If you're looking to project a confident and confident appearance, consider wearing dark shades.

Breathing

Before you start any activity, it is important to know how to breathe correctly. This article will help you understand the benefits of breathing properly.

A) to prevent illnesses (colds coughing, bronchitis, colds tuberculosis, coughing, etc.)

b) feel well

C) eliminate your lungs of pollutants as well as waste (carbon monoxide and lactic acid, etc.)

D) provide oxygen throughout thousands of cells (it is proven that deep breathing delivers 10 times more oxygen to organs)

e) combat fatigue

F) boost your energy levels

G) relax your nerves

(h) Sleep better

I) give the colour of your skin because breathing correctly improves blood circulation.

In order to increase your height, it's essential that your blood supply is oxygenated because blood provides nutrients to bones. Regular breathing also helps to cleanse your blood. The lungs are similar to balloons. When you put pressure on them, air has to go away. If not, breathing is restricted and can cause harm to you.

How do you breathe correctly while exercising

Three phases of breathing:

1. Inhaling air - breathe it into your body through your nose

2. Inhaling deeply - hold your breath within your body

3. Inhaling - blow the air in your body using your mouth

Make sure you exercise in a room that is well ventilated to ensure that you be able to breathe clean air. Each exercise should be done by breathing deeply. The graph below shows how long you can devote to each breathing phase.

INHALING, RETAINING EXHALING, AND INSTAL

4 minutes 3 seconds 12 seconds

5 seconds 3 minutes 15 seconds

6 seconds 3 minutes 12 seconds

7 seconds 3 minutes 21 seconds

Exhaling can take longer than inhaling, as it is crucial to eliminate all air out of your lungs.

Exercises to breathe

Exercises for breathing in the abdominal area will be demonstrated because it is thought to be the most effective one.

1. Laying Down

Lie down to your side and relax completely. You can place an arm on the stomach. To improve your concentration, shut your eyes. This is a relaxing exercise that will help you sleep better.

Inhale deeply by blowing your nose (you will notice your stomach filling of air).

Hold your breath.

Exhale slowly from your mouth. Your stomach will begin to deflate.

Then, contract your stomach and push out the air out of your body.

2. Standing Position

Then, raise your arms off your sides towards an upward position. in a straight line, then create an X.

Inhale the air through the nose for four seconds.

Then stretch your arms straight upwards while you breathe for 3 seconds.

Exhale slowly from the mouth, while lower your arms.

Hold your hands tightly behind your back, and then push your torso forward for 12 seconds.

• Expel all air from your lungs through tightening the stomach muscles.

Self-Back Massage

A tennis ball is a must for be used. Sit up straight in your chair. Place the tennis ball in the affected area, and then sit back. By pressing against the ball and breathing deeply, you can begin to breathe in and deep. Ten or more breaths. Repeat if necessary. Try all sorts of stretching techniques, including Yoga, Pilates or just simply reaching your feet when standing. It is important to stretch and breathe deeply for the optimal results. Cartilage is a strong but elastic material. If you do the right exercises you can stretch your cartilage to:

The vertebrae are located in the spinal column

- the thigh bones as well as,

The shin, or tibia bones.

It is possible to develop cartilage which can then create more space between the vertebrae.

If you don't exercise regularly The cartilage gets soft, and bones eventually meet and rub. The spinal column functions as an elastic coil. By stretching it upwards and down, both forwards and backwards and side-to-side it can make you more taller.

Mental Exercises

This section plays an important function in helping you to achieve your goals. It is crucial to be open and keep a close eye on this section. Your mood and mental faculties can significantly affect your size. You must have faith and believe in your own abilities that you are able to get more taller. Do not believe the books you read and what others tell you. Every morning, upon getting up from bed, you should say loudly to yourself that you've gotten larger. Each night, before you go to go to bed, remind yourself that you're about to get taller. Your mind will believe the things it believes and your body is likely respond to your thoughts. Therefore, it is essential to train your mind so you are in the best shape to get larger. Don't measure your height on a daily basis. Follow your plan and only measure it every month. You'll be surprised by how larger you've become. Your mind is a formidable thing. Researchers estimate that the majority of people use approximately 15 percent of their brain abilities. Making use of your mind is much easier than you imagine.

Guided Imagery

Guided imagery is described as the creation of images in the mind (sights or sounds and emotions) to enhance the physical and emotional healing. Positive images stimulate the nervous system, releasing neurons (chemical agents) into the bloodstream, which then reach certain cells, where they initiate healing as per Lucille Eller R.N., M.S.N. who is the principal investigator of Health Journeys HIV Guided Imagery Study at University Hospitals, Cleveland Clinic, Cleveland, Ohio.Guided imagery is known to affect heart rate blood pressure, respiration rate and body temperature, brain waves and many other. It can improve a person's general well-being and overall health or utilized to achieve specific objectives, like the growth of bones. Imagery is the first language we've ever had. When we think of memories from our past or our childhood, we think of images, images and sounds, as well as pain and so on. It's not always through words. Images aren't only visual , they can also include sounds and tastes, smells, or any combination of these. For example, a particular scent, for instance could trigger either happy or painful memories to you. It is believed that the average person is able to have 10000 thoughts, or pictures flashing in the mind daily. The majority of these thoughts are negative. Visualisations and affirmations are utilized by athletes every day. It's been proved that simply telling yourself "I can achieve this" will boost your performance by 5percent. Visualisation is a tool used by athletes to boost their performance, often without even realising that they are doing it. Be aware that it's not the object you believe to be true, rather the thought within your mind that creates the end result. Everything you experience, every event actions, conditions and experiences are created by your subconscious mind as a reaction to the thoughts you think about. Negative thoughts lead to negative experiences. Beware of untrue beliefs, superstitions or fears. If you are able to practice this, there is nothing that limits the level of improvement you can attain. Many of you might believe that it's impossible to control all thoughts that creep into your brain. It is possible to eliminate negative thoughts by using prayers or affirmations that are scientifically based. Prayer or affirmation will be granted by an universal principle of reaction and action.

Create your own mental "movie" that reflects your desired goal. Visualize what the scene would appear like when your height was 6'5" today. Imagine a memorable moment you'll have once you're taller. Then imagine it as the basis of a commercial. Concentrate intensely on the happiness in your face, then think in detail about how amazed people surrounding you will be by your new height. Make close-ups of the faces, then make the "movie" using black and white, if that is more powerful and emotional for you. Think of the most memorable emotional, most uplifting experience that you will experience once you have achieved your goal. Then, focus on it, at least three times a day, using affirmations and the belief that you can keep going.

Subconscious

The subconscious brain is a powerful capacity that has yet to fully develop to its fullest capacity. Many believe that we possess an inner spirituality and a subconscious side. It is believed that the subconscious brain and spirit are two separate entities. To fully comprehend the power of the subconscious is you need to first realize and accept it is not chance of occurrence. There is no chance that something happens. This means that everything is set in stone or planned to be.Your subconscious mind is the one that creates everything that happens in your life based on messages and information you have gave. You are

You are constantly sending messages and other messages to your mind. More than half these messages are ineffective or even harmful. And then you start to wonder why things don't improve regardless of what you do. The messages you send to your subconscious mind are the thoughts of beliefs, actions and thoughts. If you are constantly worried over not being able to afford your expenses you'll never have enough. It's that easy. If you don't believe you're capable to achieve your objectives, you'll never be able to achieve all of them. Why? Since if the information you are referring to is negative and negative, it can lead to an outcome that is negative.

Positive Thinking

Thinking positively is an aspect of living instead of a fleeting thought. It is important to think positively as an everyday habit. The concept of state of mind can be applied in a variety of ways. If you're in a positive frame of thoughts, everything appear to be better! If we're in a depressed or down mood, everything seems to get worse and worse. If you're thinking there were times you were optimistic and believed it was likely to occur and it didn'thappen? It's because you experienced doubts or affirmations that were negative. Some may be so old-fashioned or embedded into your thoughts that you might not be aware of them. It is possible to believe that your life is governed through shammy superstitions or naive affirmations, but it won't help you develop, whether physically or otherwise.

A lot of our experience is influenced on the basis of our psychological state. Let's take an example, for instance. you exercise at an exercise facility. The morning started perfectly but something that's not unusualregular routine. When you are on the treadmill you see a friend is walking over to you and asks, "You look a bit pale? We hope that you're not sick!" You've never thought about what you were feeling. You believed that you were well when you got up. In just a few minutes someone else comes up and makes the same comments.

You're sure that you aren't unwell, because many people are saying the exact similar thing! In a short period of time, you'll be feeling ill and pale! Mind is an incredibly powerful tool. If you accept someone's claim that you're short or chubby, or even annoying, will be the same impact on you like if you were. Stop thinking negative thoughts.

Relaxation Techniques

The best time to try this technique is while you're asleep and ready to sleeping. This is because you're in a state of relaxation and will be able to fall into an alpha mindwave. This makes it easier to imbue your mind with a particular goal or thought.

When you are about to go to bed Take a few minutes and "picture" something you'd like to have e.g. height! It doesn't matter whether you are able to visualize clearly but simply imagine it the best way you can. Consider your goal as if it was already happening. Make a mental movie using the techniques you learned to create in the section on mental imagery. In your "movie" thanking you for achieving your goal, or applauding your accomplishments. Take a few minutes to immerse your body in the film with all your senses as capable of including. After that, place an "frame" (white or light works) around the film to keep it contained. This signals the brain that this "movie images" is what you are trying to accomplish. Now, move the image towards the left or right depending on what your brain thinks your "past" as being. To figure out which direction you're looking for Think of something that took place prior to the present day. Pay attention to the direction in which your eyes go even if it's just slight. If it's to the right,

141

then your past is to the right and reversed. You can move your "movie" in this direction, and you're finished for the moment. Do this every evening before going to bed. You can continue the place you left off on the night before or do it again. It's recommended to start with a single film at first. This method can be used to achieve every goal you have.

Self-Hypnosis

You've probably had the experience or have a friend who has. You wake up one night and realize that your alarm clock isn't working and you must get up early the next morning. With a sense of certainty, you say you to yourself "I must get up by eightand I'll be up at 8 am." ...". The next day, you awake and it's eight o'clock.Your subconscious brain is capable of achieving its full potential. Every night , prior to falling asleep, relay positive thoughts for your mind. In order to increase your height, you can repeat the same message as before, "Everyday I am gaining in height through exercise. I am growing. "I am growing. .... ".

EXERCISES

It is widely accepted that physical exercise can stimulate the growth of bones in humans. Research has shown when you perform intense training (exercise) there is an increase of growth hormones is observed within the human body. We recommend specific time frames to adhere to when performing the exercises listed in this book We do not, however suggest doing the exercises until the extent of exhaustion. Don't overexert yourself. If you feel short of breath or feel you are becoming excessively.

The exercises we've included in this article can be completed anytime throughout the daytime. But, I don't intend for you to complete all of them in one sitting I've provided some alternatives. Pick one or two that you are comfortable doing. You can choose to do one, two, or even 10 depending on the location and when you practice them and the amount of time you'll need for these exercises. While you are doing these exercises, it will depend on when you eat and what food you take in.

Here are a few points to remember prior to working out:

1. Wear loose clothes that do not limit movement.

2. Exercises for stretching should be done in bare feet.

3. Make sure you empty your bladder and bowels prior to beginning.

4. Begin to warm up before you exercise.

5. Begin your stretching exercise slowly and smooth with a controlled approach. This is applicable to entering the position and then leaving it.

6. Do not exert yourself to the point that you are feeling discomfort. If you experience any type of exercise that makes your leg muscles feel tingly, like they're weak or numb end the exercise.

7. Relax and stretch. Only a muscle that is relaxed will allow itself to stretch.

8. Breathe comfortably and easily.

9. Be patient and persevering. Don't force or rush your self in any manner.

The exercises contained in this book will encourage the growth of your body and height and help increase the length of the spine as well as improve posture and straighten any curvature that is excessive to the spine. Through the exercise routine you'll also gain better overall health in your back and abdominal muscles, greater flexibility, as well as the relief and reduction of lower back pain.

The exercises are illustrated using simple and easy to follow instructions. The exercises are safe, efficient and simple to perform for people of all ages or fitness levels. They require no specific equipment or apparatus, and can be performed at the private space of your home.

Warming-Up

Always warm up before beginning the main exercise to ensure your body is prepared for the demands. The muscles that are warm stretch more easily and permit greater mobility for joints. Oxygen is released from blood once the muscles are slowly warmed. This helps you avoid getting exhausted early. It also enhances coordination, burns off fat more efficiently, and decreases irregular heart rhythms caused from abrupt exercise.

It will take about 15 to 20 minutes to warm up. For the first 5 to 7 minutes, you can run in a relaxed manner at a moderate pace. Remember, speed is not always more effective! You will require 10-15 minutes to get your muscles and joints. Make small leaps in one location and bend your spine with your arms firmly seated at the head's back in every direction, from the front (as as low as you can) towards the sides, and finally to rear (pic. 1, 2, 3, 4); do sit-ups (pic. 5) and curl your upper body to the left and right whilst keeping your leg in a stable position (pic. 6, 7). Then, move both arms in a horizontal direction to the back and then cross them to the front and push to the maximum extent you can. Turn your arms both vertically and try to complete it quickly (pic.8). Flex your body to the left side by lifting your left hand towards the left side with the right hand raised (pic.9 10, 10).

1 2 3 4 5 6 7 8 9 10

There are a myriad of exercises that will help you warm up your muscles and body There are exercises for each muscle. Imagine each muscle in your body and put it to work however, do not attempt something too difficult for yourself. Remember that your muscles need to be relaxed and warm rather than big and sturdy. It is important to increase your size, not muscle.

Cooling-Down

Cooling down is as crucial as warming up. This process involves return of breathing and heart rate to normal. This is extremely crucial. Begin by putting your hands in a row over your head. Then, try to get as high as you can by stretching your entire body (pic. 11). Imagine that someone attempts to drag you upwards with your hands. Try it for a minute as you walk slowly. Then, you can move your hands in a circular motion without touching one the other. Each time you raise your hands up extend your spine and legs as far as you can. Remember to not stop walking.Slow moving will stop blood from accumulating inside the legs, which could lead to dizziness or blackouts.

11

Make sure to include warm-ups as well as a cool-down portion of your workout. It is just as important as exercising in the first place, and skipping these two steps can lead to health issues. If you're doing something crucial, you must be ready to achieve great outcomes. In the event that you don't, you could ruin everything. Avoid experimenting on your health and adhere to our advice.Exercising in humid, hot or wet and cold can be difficult and dangerous. With a little preparation outdoors, exercise is enjoyable and secure at any season.Tips to exercise in hot and humidity Get plenty of water. Insufferable sweating can cause heat stroke and exhaustion. Drink plenty of fluids before, during, and following exercise , even if it doesn't feel thirsty.Use your common sense. The more greater the temperature of the air and the less humid it must be to reduce the risk of injuries from heat. In the case of temperatures rise above 80°F the risk of heat injury is high when the humidity is greater than 50 percent. In extremely humid and hot periods, you can exercise inside in the cool air or take a swim. Make sure to take time to adjust. The body requires time to adjust to temperatures that are hot. It takes between 7 and 14 days to completely acclimatize and therefore gradually increasing the amount of time you exercise.

Tips for exercising in the winter when it's rainy and cold:

Wear multiple layers of clothes. The outer layer must keep you safe from the elements like rain, wind or snow. The cold temperatures, dampness and winds increase the chance of suffering from hypothermia. It is easy to cool down the body in cold weather, and the wind can evaporate it more quickly. Wear clothing that insulates and keep out moisture. Wool and polypropylene are great as is cotton, which holds moisture.Protect particular body parts, like your face, head feet, and hands. Gloves are more comfortable than mittens. Protect your head with wool caps. Protect your face by wearing an afghan or a high collar. Use socks that will hold the heat and keep moisture out. Take plenty of water. Avoid drinking alcohol prior to or during exercise - it causes the body to lose heat more quickly. It is best to warm up inside before going outside for. By warming your muscles, you can keep you from injuries.

I don't recommend doing any exercise outdoors if the conditions are extreme. If you're a Bodybuilder or Weightlifter it is appropriate to have muscles that are strong however, not massive muscles. If you're a bodybuilder, there is a lower chance of growing at a rapid rate. If you're not planning to give up bodybuilding altogether then we suggest doing the exercises for your muscles in a slower pace. It is possible to try this at the end of your bodybuilding workout hold your muscles the longest time possible, without moving. This will make your muscles robust, but not as large. Be sure to relax your muscles following a workout

stretching, hanging from the chin-up bar and any other exercise that you are comfortable with that you can find in our training program. The majority of these exercises are great to relax muscles.

Lifting weights in a standing posture can have negative consequences for the growth of your. However the weight lifting process is extremely effective in increasing the levels of growth hormones in your blood, particularly when you lift the maximum weight. This is due to the pressure that is put on your body, which causes the release of growth hormone. To be safe it is recommended to work your chest, shoulders and arm muscles by lifting weights in the horizontal position.

The exercises listed here aren't just good to help you reach your potential for growth They are also beneficial to lose weight, keep your body in top condition, helping your heart perform better and improving your overall health in a variety of other ways.You should be doing these exercises for 4-5 days per week. It is important to not stop performing the exercises abruptly, as the program must be continuously followed in order to achieve positive results.The most effective place to exercise is outside, in a park close to you However, an exercise facility or gym is a good option in extreme weather conditions (see the section on exercising in extreme conditions).

Keep your back straight and place your feet in a broad but secure and comfortable place. Secure your hands to the rear to your neck. Your body should be bent towards your left foot, and slowly return to a standing position then bend in the middle between your legs, and then back to the straight position. then bend towards your right leg before returning to the straight position, changing at every bend. Don't move your legs in a bent position. Make sure to keep your legs straight. This may be challenging in the beginning and could be painful in the muscles in the rear of the legs. However, this is how you should do it. Do not stretch your neck too much. Try to maintain your neck straight (in one direction with the body). After every bend (left or center and right) create one turn towards the back while maintaining your balance (pic. 12). Do three sets of these gentle body bends. Next, do 5 repetitions of pushing as hard as you can. Be careful not to tighten your body, instead let it relax. Spend a minute walking. Then, do 5 more repetitions that follow the exact bends (left right, center, left) however, this time, your fingers touch with loor at each bend (pic. 13, 14, 15).

12 13 14 15

Your heart should now be pounding fast. This method is extremely efficient to slow down your heartbeat and provide additional energy to your body.

Slowly walk for a bit. Place both arms horizontally in a straight line, with your palms facing upwards so that it looks like the shape of a cross (pic. 16). Imagine a huge amount of pure energy surrounding your body. Inhale the air into your lungs, and then slowly move your arms upwards and then down before you, letting air out (pic.17 18.). As you do this, visualize that you are grabbing the energy of the outside and then putting it inside your body. Repeat this process several times until your heartbeat is lowered and you feel relaxed.

16 17 18

Keep your hands on the bar that is horizontal Relax for a few seconds, and then lift your legs and bend them towards your knees as high as you can. Maintain this position for about 20-30 seconds, then gradually lower your legs and let the bar go. Take a break for two minutes, then repeat the exercise a second time.

19

Stop for about 4-5 minutes.

Reaching jumps can be done with a the running starting. Return approximately 12-15 feet (4-5 meters) from the object you wish to reach. Begin to run slowly towards the object and make the next two steps quicker, and then leap while pulling up using both feet as well as stretching your legs towards the object with your hands. Repeat these jumps five times. After some time then repeat them 10 times, using only the same leg, changing the direction from right to left and back every time.

These are the essential steps that you should perform every day, at least 4-5 times per week (as I mentioned earlier). I'll give you additional details about these exercises: If plan to perform these exercises with someoneelse, you could ask your partner to keep your feet in place when you're hanging from the bar that is horizontal, however the person holding you should not pull your feet too strongly.Another technique is to make sure that while you're hanging off bars, you companion standing on a stool is supposed to place his hands over your hands to assist you in avoiding fall off the bar, and also to hold long enough. This method is extremely useful for those who don't have enough strength in their hands to hold themselves on the bars for an extended period of time (mostly women, children, and women fall into that category).).

As I mentioned earlier the most ideal location to exercise in the morning is outside, maybe in the park.

Fresh and clean air is the ideal setting to maximize the results of this exercise. It will make your blood full of oxygen, and this will provide plenty of energy to your body. It will not only allow you increase your growth rate however, it will provide you with fresh air that enhances the health of each aspect of your body, and your mind.

If you plan to exercise at home, you must first ensure that you have plenty of space within your house and that there are no neighbors who are disturbed. Also, ensure that there's no furniture to fall off while you perform leaps. Here's the information you'll require...

In the beginning, you must have an upright bar installed in your home. This will be your primary exercise equipment. Wherever you perform your workout, you'll require an horizontal bar in your home. It's a specially-designed bar specifically designed for home use. It can be hung in between vertical walls (walls) which are located close to one another or on the door frame. It should be sufficiently high to ensure that your feet don't be in contact with the floor when you sit your bar. Remember, you'll grow taller, and in the future, you could become too tall for the bar's height. The distance between your feet to your flor when hanging should be between 4 and 7 inches.

The window should be opened. You require fresh air, and your blood requires oxygen. The indoor fitness program is nearly the same as the outdoor one. The only difference is that you may not have enough space to do jumping and running, except if you have a home gym that has a track for running or this exercise at the nearby fitness centre.

If you do not have enough space for an outdoor event Here's a different option:

While you're warming up you could skip the slow running and perform easy, relaxed jumping instead. A treadmill is an excellent piece of fitness equipment, as it is slow-paced running that can be the best exercise to keep your health in good condition. To achieve the goals we're aiming for it's not required to own this type of apparatus.

Running is a great method to get ready for the primary exercise. You could also substitute distance running by running in the same place (continuous light joggingthat keeps your legs moving). A indoor object that could be used in place of the tree branches could be any object with a high-overhang that is only accessible through jumping, like a ceiling or a piece of cloth which is high enough that it's difficult to reach.

Since you're at home, you are able to exercise in ways that aren't usually possible to exercise outside. These two exercises are great for stretching your legs, back and abdominal muscles. All of these areas that are crucial to your body's capacity to grow.

Lay down on your floor (preferably on the floor) and place your legs close together and straight ahead behind the you (do not bend your knees). Place your hands underneath your calves as high as you are able to reach, and then push your body toward your legs, pushing hard enough that you feel a bit of discomfort on your calves. Keep this position for 2 minutes, and then release. Repeat this four times. Then, repeat it while pressing your body to the maximum extent you can for 20-30 minutes. Place your body on the floor on your back and then rest for one minute (pic. 20, 21).

20 21

Place your feet on the floor , with your face towards the floor. Put your feet on the ground underneath the shoulders (pic. 22). Slowly raise your arms and straighten them, lift the upper part of your body from of the floor. Then, raise your back. The lower part of your body must be in a relaxed state (pic. 23). Your head must rise as much as is feasible. Keep this position for about 4 to 5 minutes. Repeat the exercise 3 times, pushing harder each time.

time.

22

23

Place your feet on the floor, with your legs in a straight line. Lean your body toward your toes and try to reach them. It is important to not move the legs (pic. 24).

24

The exercises mentioned above are a crucial component of getting taller, but it isn't enough to get the best outcomes. It is important to realize that growth is a continuous process. In order to encourage your body to develop, you must to work out constantly.

When you are standing Place your hands on your head, and then interlock your fingers. Make use of your arm and hand muscles for pushing your head up and backwards, while simultaneously using the neck muscles in order to counter the pushing motion. When you are applying these pressures and allowing your head to be pulled up until your head is resting upon your chest. Let the pressure off your head and then bring it back to its normal position. Repeat the process 10 times, and then take a break for 10 seconds and repeat the procedure 10 times more. (pic.25,26)

25 26

When you are standing with your head elevated, arms to your sides. Move your arms backwards and lock with your fingers behind you back and below your waist. This is the starting point. While keeping your thumbs locked, and your arms as straight as they can be and bring your shoulders upwards and back down, and then forward, then upwards then back, down, forward, executing an arc and trying to stretch your shoulders as much as is possible in all directions. Do this exercise slowly, always mindful that you're stretching your shoulders to the limit. Do three rounds of 10 circular movements. You can take a brief time during each round. (pic.27,28)

27 28

When you are standing, with your arms extended horizontally from the body. Rotate the arms around about 2 feet in diameter. Maintain the arms at a 45 degree angle, and don't bend your elbows. Turn the arms away in your shoulder joint. After a few rotations, turn your arms to the other direction a few times. The arms should be extended as far as they can with each rotation. (pic.29)

29

The following actions are essential...

Physical Activity in the course of the day

Your posture

It is important to alter your posture and stand, and how you walk. As you read this article, pay close focus on your posture. Are you bending your neck slightly and trying to support your head in a slack position, or do you hold your head straight? What about your spine? Do you have a straight spine or does it appear like the shape of a question mark? Do you see what I am talking about? Yes, this is crucial to your health. The spinal disks need to be under minimum pressure A way to lessen the stress for your back is to ensure your back is straight throughout the day.

Imagine the body you are growing extremely quickly. Begin to slowly stretch your entire body upwards, making appear as if you're growing an inch in a matter of minutes. Try to lift your head on the highest point you can. Keep this posture for a short time and then relax, while maintaining the same posture. This is the pose you need to maintain throughout your life. It not only makes more easy for the body develop This position of your body can prevent many illnesses in the near future. Your brain can also function better when you sit in this position. Additionally, it's difficult to fatigue standing straight up.

Another option to determine the ideal posture best suited to your physique is to remain on the wall, securing the wall by your shoulders, back and head. The shoulders should be spread out, but not too much to cause discomfort.

In the course of the day regardless of what you do, you should stretch your body whenever you feel like it. Make your body grow and be sure to do it correctly. Imagine your body growing immediately and then try to feel it.

Jumps

We don't advise doing jumps one hour before and after meals, or one hour prior to bed. You can choose any time to do them, whether at home, reaching for the ceiling, outside-reaching to branches of trees or any other object. A fitness center is an ideal place to practice jumps. It is recommended to perform 200-300 jumps per day. Volleyball or basketball is the most effective method to achieve your goal of jumping. If you can exceed 300 jumps, the more. The importance of jumping is in getting the most growth possible.

Floor Exercises

Knees-to chest hug: Lie down on your back, then bring your knees together and place them on your chest. From there you can wrap the arms of your legs, then pull your knees toward your chest, while at all times, pulling your chin towards your chest. Repeat the exercise twice, holding the position for 15 to 20 minutes (pic.30)

30

Knees to the side Place your body on your back with your with your knees bent, and your feet lying flat on the floor. Let the legs drop onto one side. Then, let the legs drop to the side on the opposite. Each time, hold the position for 10 second (pic. 31).

31

Leg and arm opposite on stomach: Lay down face-down in the ground. From there then raise your left arm as well as your right leg to the highest you can (pic.32). For 3-4 seconds, hold the position and then return to the ground gradually. Repeat the same exercise using your left and right arms. Repeat these 10 times. Then relax by lying in a position on your floor for a minute.

32

Leg and opposite arm sitting on knees: Get on all fours and rest on your knees and hands. Your eyes should be straight down and keep your head parallel to the body. From there then, raise and straighten your right leg and left arm until they are in line with the ground , or greater (as as high as you can). Do this for 3-4 minutes before coming back slowly to your starting position. Repeat the exercise with the left and right arms.

Five repetitions per side are sufficient for novices, and 10 times on a regular routine (pic. 33).

33

Your knees and hands are on the floor: Keep on all foursand place the majority the weight of your body on knees. Moving your body to your hands, perform one push-up and then step back to the maximum distance you can by attempting to sit up on your feet. Finally, get returning to push-ups repeatedly 15 to 20 times. Your hands should remain in the same position every time. Push-ups aren't only a fantastic way to strengthen your chest, arms or back muscles. They also strengthen your heart, and fill your bloodstream with oxygen as well as growth hormone. It is possible to work on

Different muscles place your hands in different distances from each another and at different angles(pic.34)

34

Elongation: Lie flat on your back with arms extended fully above your head. and legs fully extended on the floor. stretch your body all the way from your fingertips all the way to your toes, extending your body both ways. In this position, turn your body's upper part to the left, and then to the right, while maintaining your hips on the floor. This is a great exercise to do when you're lying in bed.Before getting up every morning (and before you go to bed every evening) Stretch your legs and arms until the limit. Place your toes at the bottom of your bed. Then, then point your arms out to the headboard of your bed and extend your body until it is stretched to the limit. Turn and twist your body in every direction possible by stretching each joint and muscle of the body simultaneously.(pic. 35).

35

In the in a prone position, lying flat on your back, with your arms close to your sides Lift your arms up and straighten them to your head until they're extended onto the floor and pointing toward your face. With all you weight onto your stretched arms, shoulders, and on your heels slowly lift your back and hips, the torso, and your upper legs off the floor. Then, stretch your body as high as you are able to. Maintain the position for a couple of secondsbefore returning to your original position. Repeat the exercise five times. (pic.36,37)

36 37

The effects of heat and water

An effective method to stimulate growth zones is to use the sauna or a warm bath. If you're taking bath it is recommended that it is recommended that the bath should be between 98 and 102 degrees (37C-39C). Add sea salt to warm water and then stay there the time you are comfortable in the bathing water. Make sure to do this prior to going to bed. This will increase the metabolism of your body, and allows your body to respond faster to changes in your physical activity.

Participate in recreational activities

It will be helpful in assisting this particular program we've developed for you, if you take part in as many leisure activities as your schedule allows. Get involved in various sporting organizations within your local community. All extra activities can aid in the growth of bone in your body, which is an added benefit along with the exercises we recommend. If you're choosing an sport, you should select one that will give you the greatest benefits towards increasing your height. In other words, choose an activity that provides your torso and legs with the chance to stretch out and active. Some good examples of these types of activities include swimming, tennis or basketball, racquetball gymnastics, aerobics, etc.

Chapter 13: "Eat The Right Kinds Of Food

"The food you consume can be either the most safe and most potent form of medicine or the most slow type that poison."

- Ann Wigmore

The height we attain is mostly determined by our genes , however it also depends on the foods we consume, especially during the growth times. If we consume the right types of food then we are likely to attain our height to the maximum. In contrast in the event that we are deficient in certain nutrients our development could be slowed. The primary nutrient that allows our body's development is protein. Protein is considered to be the component of our skeletal system, which includes cartilages, bones, and tissues. The skeletal system is the body with a frame in which the weight of muscle and fat is included in.

It is crucial to eat sufficient amounts of protein throughout our developing years to help us achieve our height maximum. However, as we attempt to increase our intake of foods that are rich in protein We must be aware of foods that have a high amount of fats and carbohydrates. A high intake of fats and carbohydrates can hinder the process of proteins, and consequently hinder the growth rate.

The protein-rich food items you can include in your diet routine are oatmeal, skimmed dairy eggs, soybeans, eggs chicken and meat. It is also recommended to make sure that your daily intake also includes other food groups that assist in developing your body. You should ensure that you consume sufficient amounts of meat, fruits vegetables, grains, as well as healthy fats. Make sure to choose high-quality foods to ensure you're not ingesting poisonous ingredients and other toxins that could hinder the growth of your body. It is also beneficial to increase your intake of calcium because calcium is essential in the growth of bones. In order for calcium to absorb into your body, you must to make sure that you're receiving enough vitamin D.

Vitality of Vitamins

Vitamins can be considered among the crucial elements in ensuring the highest height growth as well as maintaining an overall healthy body. Out of all the nutrients are required to consume, Vitamin D can be thought of as the most vital not just to promote growth, but also for maintaining strong bones, too. In case you are looking to grow to your highest height it is crucial to eat high-quality vitamin D foods regularly. A few of the foods high in vitamin D are potatoes, cauliflower, tomatoes and various citrus fruits. If you eat these food items regularly to be able to prevent vitamin deficiencies which could cause growth slowing.

Another vital vitamin must be consumed to boost your growth potential includes Vitamin B1. A few of the food items that are high in Vitamin B1 include peanuts rice, pork as well as soybeans, beans and soya beans. Vitamin B1 isn't just used to assist in growing, but helps in the that the digestive, cardiovascular and nervous systems.

Vitamin B2 is also known as riboflavin is crucial in ensuring optimal height growth. It is available in sources like eggs, fish as well as green leafy vegetables, and milk.

Also, make sure you have adequate quantities in Vitamin C in order to make sure that the muscles and bones develop in a healthy way. It is possible to get Vitamin C from potatoes, tomatoes, berries and the majority of citrus fruits.

The importance of Zinc and Minerals

Apart from foods that are vitamin-rich it is also important to include foods that are rich in zinc and other minerals into your daily diet to help you grow to your highest height. The most vital minerals must be avoided from being deficient in include fluoride, zinc manganese, iodine, and calcium. Calcium is essential for the development and maintaining strong bones. it is typically located in dairy items, particularly milk.

The foods that are high with minerals comprise collards spinach, turnips and the majority of soy-based food items. Research has shown that the consumption of zinc-rich foods may help in increasing the height of a person. The zinc-rich food items include eggs, yeast as well as lamb, peanuts dried watermelon seeds, steak oysters, and pumpkin seeds. Zinc is not just vital to ensure maximum growth, but it also plays a significant role in increasing the metabolism of your body.

Iodine is a different mineral that aids in increasing growth. If you ensure that you have an sufficient amounts of iodine within your body, you'll not only be able to ensure the highest growth but also make sure the thyroid gland is working well and that the other body's parts are developing correctly. A few of the foods that are enriched with iodine include cereals, fish tomatoes, meat and green peas.

Do you require supplements to increase your the size of your body?

As we have discussed it is important to make sure that you get enough amounts of proteins, fats minerals, carbohydrates and vitamins in your daily diet to guarantee maximum growth. Many people are unable to find or prepare food that has the recommended daily allowance of every one of the essential nutrients. This is the reason diet supplements are now available on the market. But, prior to deciding to purchase and consume any food supplements, talk to your physician to make sure that you're not taking supplements that could cause harm rather than positive effects. There are certain hormone supplements and medicines that assist in stimulating the growing glands in the human body. If used correctly or according to the prescription, these supplements will increase your height by a few inches. However, you don't really require these advanced supplements. It is enough to make sure that you are getting enough in calcium as well as Vitamin D within your normal diet - whether by taking supplements or natural foods. A lot of people do not remember to increase their Vitamin D which renders their calcium intake useless.

*) Get to your height maximum potential by feeding your body with adequate amounts of the vital nutrients it requires.

Start a regular exercise routine

" To experience the glow of fitness, you need to work out."

- Gene Tunney

It is no doubt that height plays a crucial aspect in the development of the person's appearance. This is the reason so many people are looking for ways to increase their height in every possible way. Due to the increasing popularity, we are able to discover a myriad of Acupressure treatments as well as other medicines which claim to work in boosting a person's height. But, before shelling out your hard-earned cash to purchase these costly treatments, it is important to be sure to thoroughly evaluate their efficacy. Be aware of the negative unwanted side effects that these treatments typically come with. It is not advisable to put your health in danger with treatments that can't ensure 100% efficiency.

Before looking for synthetic methods to boost your height, it's recommended to explore natural options like regular exercise routines that are accompanied by a healthy eating habits and nutrition. If you exercise regularly you'll not only increase the chances of reaching your height and potential, but you'll also be in a position to tone and build your muscles while maintaining an active and healthy body. Remember to combine fitness with a healthy nutrition to ensure the fresh and active growth hormones as well as to build and strengthen your muscles.

While it's generally accepted we are in large part determined by genetics but we can still take certain things like exercising and eating habits to increase the chances of achieving our maximum height potential. Most of us end our growth after the beginning of adolescence as a result of the joining between the plates of growth inside the long bones of the body. But, it's possible to keep growing and to gain some inches when you're in your 20s, if you follow certain exercises that promote the height of your body.

To get the most effective outcomes, try and do the following exercises 2 to three times a week. Be sure to avoid over-training as exercising too much can cause injuries and eventually cause growth to be slowed.

Bar Leaping

Have you ever thought that gravity could make you appear shorter due to the fact that it compresses spine and joints, which then reduces and compresses cartilage? One of the most effective and most efficient ways to tackle this issue is to hang from a bar that is vertical. If hanging from the bar you permit the lower portion of your body to lengthen your spine, which reduces the force exerted upon your vertebra. This could lead to an increase in height of one or two inches. Don't believe that height increases can be seen after just one workout. It is important to remain patient and do this exercise regularly.

The bar is used to perform this exercise should be set at a level where you are able to let your body extend while still having enough room to move. If it's not possible to get the bar that can allow your body to fully extend and extend, then simply move your knees, so you can still remain in a position to move freely. Be sure you're secure in your grip on the bar and ensure that the hand palms are facing outward towards. While hanging on the bar, ensure that your arms, shoulders and hips are at a comfortable level. This allows gravity to pull your body down. To increase the pulling force, you may choose to use ankle weights.

It is recommended to hang free on the bar for approximately twenty seconds. Take a break after which you can continue repeating at least three or four times. In the list of exercises proven to improve the height of a person, bar hanging is thought as the one most efficient.

Dry Land Swim

Swimming on dry land is frequently referred to as alternate Kicking. The primary focus of this exercise is the lower back.

For the first time lay down on your stomach lying flat on a mat or on the floor. Be sure your body is fully stretched. Set both your arms on the floor in front of you. Make sure that your palms of your hands are facing downwards to the floor. Slowly lift your right arm over the left arm. Make sure that both legs are straight. While doing this move one leg off the floor as far off the ground as you are able to. Maintain this position for no less than four seconds. Follow the same procedure using your left arm and right leg. Your goal is to maintain this posture for at least 20 minutes.

If you're looking to boost the effects of this workout it is possible to put on wrist and ankle weights, which will increase the resistance and strengthen the muscles of the lower back.

Pelvic Shift

Despite the simple nature of this exercise, it's extremely efficient for giving your body an excellent up and down stretch using your spine and hips.

For the first time lay down on your back resting on the floor or mat. Set your shoulders and arms comfortably onto the floor. Bend both knees while keeping both of the feet close to each other as is possible. Next, you must raise your back, allowing you to push your pelvis to an upward direction. You should keep this posture for 20-30 minutes. When you regularly practice this exercise you'll be able to stretch your muscles and increase the flexibility of your hips. flexible.

Cobra Stretch

The aim of this exercise is to provide your spine with a nice stretch that will eventually increase its flexibility and make it flexible. This particular workout is effective in allowing your cartilages between the vertebrae to develop. The result is a rise in height.

For this exercise, lay down on the floor or on a mat with your face facing downwards. Place the palms of both arms resting on the floor directly below your shoulders. Your spine should be fully arching until your chin is to the top of your chin. It is possible to arch as high as you like, however, each time you attempt this exercise, you should aim to return your arch a bit further. Try this exercise for at least three to four times. Maintain the position for 5 to 30 seconds before taking a break.

Super Cobra Stretch

For this exercise, lay down on a mat the floor with your head down and both of your hands on the floor beneath your shoulders. Then, fully arch your spine until your chin is to the highest point. Now, bend your hips in such a way that you can allow your body to move into an upside-down V-position. When you are stretching ensure that your chin is securely placed against your chest. Maintain the position for 10 to twenty seconds , then return to your original posture and relax.

Hopping on One Leg

This is another easy exercise that can be done almost anyplace. This exercise can be done while you watch your favorite TV show , you are watching your children play at the park, or as you do the other chores around the house.

Simply jump on your right leg eight times, while maintaining your hands in a downward direction. Then, repeat similar exercises on the left leg. The bounce motion helps not just for activating growth hormones as well as in forming your brain as well as strengthening your legs and.

Pilates Roll Over

This is a great exercise that will aid to give your spine a stretching exercise. It also gives your upper body more length. Another benefit of performing it is the vertebrae in your neck will be stretched and lengthened.

To start this exercise, lie down on mats or on the ground with your body to the floor, and your arms between your legs. Make sure that your palms of hands are facing downwards. Keep your legs together and increase the length until they are straight and pointed towards the ceiling. Bend your legs inwards until they touch the mat. It is possible that touching the mat or floor in this way may be difficult initially. However, when you keep practicing this technique it will become more comfortable. Remember that as you do stretching exercises and exercises, your spine will be lengthened and more flexible.

Forward Spine Stretch

For the first time to begin, lie on a mat, with the back straight, and with your legs ahead of you. Be sure your legs are fully extended. Your legs should be separated by at minimum the width of your shoulders. When you breathe and out, stretch both your arms forward. While you breathe, gradually turn your body forward and continue to stretch your arms until they are able to touch your toes. When you stretch your arms in by bending your arms in this manner, you are creating a flex in your spine at its highest point. If you're not able to bend enough to reach your toes, that's okay. Simply try reaching the maximum distance you can. While you continue to do the exercises for flexibility your body will get more flexible.

Cat Stretch

This exercise for flexibility is known as"the Indian Dandwat. The goal for this workout is to aid to open your spine, while strengthening your shoulders, back palms, chest and back. As you work out you'll stretch your hamstrings, while applying pressure to the stomach region. This exercise can be effective in improving blood circulation.

For the first time begin by placing your knees, as well as your hands onto a mat or the floor. Make sure both arms are locked. Breathe in as you bend your spine downwards, then exhale while you raise your back and then bring your head downwards. Now, you should arch your spine as high as you can, while making sure your elbows are aligned and shoulders up. At this point your pelvic bone at a level with the floor. Repeat the exercise 10 to 12 times , with each session lasting from three to eight seconds.

The Bow Down

To begin the exercise start by standing straight and placing your hands on your hips. As you remain in this upright in a straight line, slowly bend your body forwards as far as you are able to. Be sure that your head is in the direction of the forward bend. However, keep on your toes that they must stay straight and locked. While you're bent down ensure that your chin isn't over your chest. Repeat this process three to five times, with each set lasting between up or eight seconds.

Forward Bend

It is a well-known and widely followed stretching exercise, which is believed for its ability to boost the height of your body. To begin make sure you stand straight, making sure your legs are wide apart. When you're sitting in this posture, you can extend upwards your hands, keeping them straight. Slowly bend your arms until you're at the floor with your hands. However, make sure your knees do not bend. After three seconds, you can go back to your starting position.

Spot Jump

For the first time start by standing straight and maintaining your legs close. After that, slowly raise your body until you're sitting on the floor. Start the jump with your hands straightened upwards. You should continue to jump for at least 2 minutes.

Hands on the Bow of the Head Down

For the first time start by standing up and placing your hands on the back of your neck. Slowly bend to the side as far as you are able to. Then bend until your chin touches your chest, but ensure that your knees do not remain bent. Repeat the sequence 3 to 5 times , with each session lasting about four to eight seconds. If you are unable to touch your chest at this point, keep trying. Keep in mind the fact that flexibility is going to increase by the time you keep doing the exercises.

Super Stretch

For the first time start by standing up and placing both hands on the back of your neck. Slowly bend your head to the lowest point you are able to. Repeat the exercise 3 to 5 times , with each cycle lasting between five to 15 minutes.

Wall Stretch

To begin start by standing in a straight position with your back to the wall. Lift your hands until they are the highest you can. While doing this, you could choose to raise your body until you're sitting on your feet. Be sure your spine remains straight against the wall. The entire cycle should run about four to six seconds. Some believe that this exercise is easy , however it could be quite

Conclusion

This is all I wanted to say today. I hope that you find it informative and helpful. As I mentioned it's the program that has worked for me and I highly recommend. Surprisingly, it's easy to learn and won't take any effort.

It's still possible to gain by a few inches even if your teenage years and childhood long ago. This guide is meant for everyone to follow because it is applicable to everyone. This program was created to help you gain about 4 inches over the course of two months. There are variations depending on your body's structure and dedication.

I am unable to make any commitments to you as everything is dependent on your willingness to commit and your the free will of you. But I can say that I've done my best in my power to convey the information as precisely as is possible... in addition to being as easy as it is. I am confident that this guide will provide you with high-quality assistance but only if you require it and would like it.

You've learned more about how your body functions. You've discovered more about the activities happening in your body while you're reading this article. You've discovered how you can utilize this information to your advantage to increase your height. It sounds like a great idea isn't it?

There's no way to express the joy that comes from the achievement. It was a struggle changing my sleep habits and organising my busy life and eating well, working out daily and choosing reliable friends. However, in the end it's all worth it. I guarantee it.

Why do people prefer taller people? Why is it that height could be a barrier to the job you want in certain instances? Where has the enchantment of the mignonettes gone in a flash? Why do certain couples draw all of the awkward stares when they're taller than them?

www.ingramcontent.com/pod-product-compliance
Lightning Source LLC
Chambersburg PA
CBHW060328030426
42336CB00011B/1253